THE EMT REVIEW MANUAL

Self-Assessment Practice Tests for Basic Life Support Skills

Fourth Edition

Donald J. Ptacnik

W.B. SAUNDERS COMPANY
A Division of Harcourt Brace & Company
Philadelphia   London   Toronto   Montreal   Sydney   Tokyo

W.B. SAUNDERS COMPANY
A Division of
Harcourt Brace & Company

The Curtis Center
Independence Square West
Philadelphia, Pennsylvania 19106

Dedication
To Timothy J. Ward, who persuaded when I needed persuasion, who stood by when I needed support, and who screamed and shouted when I needed a little more persuasion. Without his constant guidance and support, this book would have been little more than a forgotten conversation. "You had to be there." (J.B.)

Copyright © 1993 by W. B. Saunders Company

Manufactured in the United States of America. All rights reserved. No portion of this book may be reproduced in any form or by any means without written permission of the publisher.

International Standard Book Number: 0-7216-5043-0

9 8 7 6 5 4 3 2

In the writing of this review manual, the author and publisher have made every attempt to follow current practices in prehospital emergency care. Suggested drug selections and dosages conform to current protocols at the time of publication. Treatment techniques are reviewed with equal concern for the most uniformly accepted protocols and procedures. It is the responsibility of the reader to conform to local standards and to be aware of new research conclusions, technological advancements, and government regulations that dictate changes which may alter suggested drug therapies or treatment protocols.

Preface

For some time, you have been studying emergency medical technology. Now you face an important challenge—scoring sufficiently high on your EMT examinations to qualify for EMT certification.

Understanding the objective of each exam will assist you through your training course, certification examinations, and later recertification exams. The written exam is designed to test your cognitive knowledge. Do you know terminology, anatomy, diagnosis, etc.? The practical exam is a little more complex. It does, of course, test your psychomotor skills, but it also evaluates your cognitive knowledge. Together the two exams call for sound decision-making abilities and practical skills demonstrated in a given period of time.

The purpose of this review manual is to develop your confidence to pass the written and practical certification exams you will take at the end of an EMT course. The manual will also act as an excellent resource for EMTs as they prepare for the examinations of the National Registry or recertification exams that are now required by many states. Also, the manual will provide knowledge and confidence required when the EMT is "on the street."

To accomplish these goals, this review manual uses multiple-choice questions and answers with meaningful rationale. Using the manual during an EMT course will reinforce material contained in your textbooks, knowledge gained during lectures, and application of the psychomotor skills on which the EMT relies so heavily. The competent EMT must combine all of this knowledge in order to provide effective patient care. The strength of the EMT is developed through understanding a patient's assessment, and then, knowing what to do or what not to do, when to do it (many activities seem to occur almost simultaneously), how fast it must be done, and most importantly WHY it needs to be done.

Since 1977, I have developed and written certification exams (written and practical) for use at the state levels. During the same period, I administered thousands of practical exams and one issue became clear. The weakness of the students was in knowing WHY they were doing a particular task. Of course, we are considering a more complex level than "Question: Why do CPR? Answer: To save lives." The many details that you must recall and perform during your initial patient examination, treatment, and re-examination have a multitude of fine components. Through the use of this review manual, you will start to manage all of these components, building from simple to complex, until you possess the knowledge and confidence to face the certification exams and the real test, the patient.

If you, as an EMT, remember the "whys" while performing your skills, you will be much less likely to make errors. The solid basis from which you then develop confidence will be unshattered when you are confronted with the complex multiple systems trauma patient or the certification/recertification exams.

Acknowledgments

I wish to thank the following individuals for their helpful comments and suggestions regarding the manuscript: Mark Stevens, EMT-P (Buck Medical Services, Portland, OR); Michael Somes, EMT-P (EMS consultant, Apple Valley, MN); and Mary Ann Talley, BSN, MPA (University of South Alabama/EMS Education, Mobile, AL).

Christopher Smith, the project coordinator, has continued to provide me with expert guidance during the preparation of this and the other review manuals I have prepared. His experience in publishing similar books for the nursing profession and advanced EMT levels has helped thousands of students nationwide to efficiently prepare for licensure exams. It remains our combined hope that this review manual will assist you during the examination process and the future application of these lifesaving skills.

Contents

1. The Art of Effective Test Taking 1
2. Roles and Responsibilities of the EMT 17
3. Personal Safety 27
4. Anatomy, Physiology, and Diagnostic Signs 37
5. Respiratory and Circulatory Systems 61
6. Wounds, Bleeding, and Shock 101
7. Musculoskeletal System 133
8. Nervous System and Head Injuries 155
9. Chest, Abdominal, and Genital Injuries 169
10. Medical Emergencies 187
11. Childbirth and Pediatric Emergencies 217
12. Environmental Injury Emergencies 237
13. Behavioral Problems 255

14. Transportation, Patient Handling, and Scene Management 267

15. Situational Reviews 283

    Critical Questions 315

    Bibliography 317

Introduction

The purpose of this manual is to assist you in preparing more effectively for your certification and recertification exams. An effective preparation cycle will include reviewing EMT content, testing yourself to confirm strong areas and to identify your weak ones and, finally, getting yourself mentally prepared to take these important examinations.

The EMT Review Manual will assist you in analyzing your strengths and weaknesses in each EMT subject area. Over 750 questions have been included to closely simulate the types of questions appearing on Basic Life Support EMT certification exams being administered across the nation today. The manual has been organized into fifteen chapters which allows it to be used in concert with initial EMT training courses or as a free-standing review guide. Each chapter builds your knowledge, starting with simple principles and moving to the more complex. This format makes the manual an excellent review guide for the already certified EMT, as you can select individual human systems for review and study.

The manual is more than just a series of multiple-choice questions and answers. Each answer is accompanied by supporting rationale (a reasoned exposition of principles). A thorough review of each rationale will reinforce your learning by describing the underlying principle of the answer selected as correct. The rationale often goes on to explain or define the remaining three answers which provides you with additional learning experience. It should be noted that the answers selected as correct are based on nationally accepted standards and may not always be consistent with your own local training or treatment protocols.

Chapter 1, The Art of Effective Test Taking, was designed especially for the student preparing for EMT certification. Subjects in this section include helpful strategies such as how to understand questions, how to eliminate distractors, how to recognize the four basic question types, how to review, and how to maximize your test-taking effectiveness.

The following guidelines are offered in order that you may maximize your potential for learning through the use of this manual:

1. Complete one chapter at a time allowing yourself approximately one minute to answer each question.

2. Review each answer and its rationale. You will receive positive reinforcement for your correct answers and explanation for incorrect answers.

3. Determine those topic areas in which you are weak and review your text or seek additional instruction. A list of critical questions follows Chapter 15. Should you answer any of these questions incorrectly, extra review on that specific topic is indicated. A bibliography is also provided listing several excellent references.

4. As a caution, keep in mind that the questions in this manual are representative of the type of questions which appear on certification exams, but are not necessarily a "standard" examination.

5. Re-read Chapter 1 (The Art of Effective Test Taking) the day before you take your certification exams.

1 The Art of Effective Test Taking

Introduction

Knowing how to take tests is an art that is developed and enhanced through experience and by allowing one's inner creativity to be expressed. This chapter discusses the art of test taking because knowing how to take a test is almost as important as having the basic knowledge and information necessary to answer the questions correctly. Your EMT education will have provided you with the basic knowledge. This chapter and the ones following will enable you to apply this information to test-taking in the most efficient way. Then, when you sit for certification exams, you will have not only the basic information, but also the inner confidence and test-taking ability that will allow you to score well on either the state or National Registry examination.

Test-taking ability can be divided into three categories: mastery of basic knowledge and information; awareness of test-taking techniques and strategies; and, finally, freedom from anxiety that, if present at a high level, will interfere with application of both of the other categories.

State certification examinations are minimal competency exams. The exam that you will be taking is not designed to test your total knowledge, your expert ability to function in the field, or even your degree of professionalism. Its purpose is to test **whether or not you are able to function at a safe practitioner level**. It is important to keep in mind that these questions are designed to test if you can recall key EMT knowledge, assess critical situations and make proper judgments, choose appropriate EMT interventions, and, finally, recognize and select among EMT priorities.

State and National Registry written examinations are multiple-choice tests. Each question is constructed so that one of the four alternatives is the correct answer. It is important that you, the student, understand the construction and intent of the question so that you will be able to apply your knowledge in choosing the one correct answer. In the following sections, basic principles of test-taking strategy will be described.

Understanding the Question

The question is called the **stem**, and the answer choices are called **distractors**. The purpose of distractors is to distract you from identifying and choosing the correct answer. Thus, in the process of taking a multiple-choice test, all of your knowledge, expertise, and judgment are utilized.

Principle 1

In effective test construction (and we have to assume that your EMT exam is based on principles of good test construction), the stem is direct and to the point. This means that the question is asking for one particular response and that you should **not** read other information into the question. Often, you will find questions that are asking for "common sense" answers. Reading into these questions or searching for subtle hidden meanings is not advised. *Principle: Do not read extra meaning into the question; assume it is direct and to the point.* Your first action then, upon being presented with the question, is to ask yourself "What is this question asking?" Look for key words or phrases to help you understand. It is important to have the central point clearly in your mind before going on to consider the distractors.

Principle 2

Make very sure you read the stem correctly. Notice particularly the way the question is phrased. Is it asking for the **right** or the **wrong** response? Is it requiring that you choose one exception to EMT actions? Is it asking you for factual information, conceptual information, or EMT judgment? One of the most important principles in test taking is understanding what the question is asking. *Principle: Understand exactly what the stem is asking before considering the distractors.*

> *Example Question:* EMT care for a patient suffering from hemorrhagic shock includes all of the following except:

A. Controlling obvious bleeding.
B. Preventing loss of body heat.
C. Elevating lower extremities.
D. Administering low-concentration oxygen.

The question (stem) is asking you to identify the one incorrect response. There will be three correct and one incorrect alternatives. If you are reading the stem too quickly or if your anxiety level is too high, you may miss the key word "*except*," thus answering the question incorrectly. D is the correct answer. A, B, and C would all be correct EMT actions. D is an incorrect EMT action because it would be important to administer a high concentration of oxygen to the patient in shock, since the blood supply available to carry oxygen is greatly reduced, resulting in inadequate perfusion of tissues, and leading to death.

Let us look at another example of test question construction. This question is asking you to choose an EMT action that does **not usually** occur. In order to answer this question correctly, you must determine the condition that may, but does not usually, occur.

> *Example Question:* Patients with diabetes mellitus may develop acute emergency conditions known as diabetic coma and insulin shock. Which of the following signs does not usually occur in diabetic coma (ketoacidosis)?

Before considering the distractors, understand the stem. What is the question asking? First, it is asking about the diabetic coma, which is different from insulin shock. If you miss this essential point, you will not choose the correct answer. Second, the question is asking for the condition that does **not usually** occur.

A. Air hunger, rapid and deep respirations.
B. Full, rapid pulse.
C. Sweet or fruity odor on breath.
D. Excessive loss of body water.

The correct answer is B. During the condition of diabetic coma, the pulse is usually weak and rapid. The loss of body fluid, also known as hypovolemia, will result in increased pulse rate and lower blood pressure as in other states of shock. To choose the correct answer, you should have drawn two separate conclusions: the stem is asking for a particular characteristic of diabetes mellitus, and it is asking for a condition that does not usually occur.

Principle 3

Another technique for assessing the stem and interpreting the question correctly is to rephrase the question so that it is very clear in your own mind. For example, consider the following statement: "The one treatment that is not required in cardiogenic shock is . . ." Rephrase it to read: "They are asking me to identify a treatment that is not required in cardiogenic shock, but may be required in other shock conditions." Rephrasing in your own language can assist you to read the question correctly and, in turn, choose the appropriate response. This is particularly important when you are faced with a difficult and/or confusing question.

> *Example Question:* The EMT at the scene of an automobile accident is unable to perform CPR; he meets with airway resistance each time he attempts ventilation. An obstruction is suspected. Other conditions important for the EMT to note are which of the following?

To better understand the question, restate the condition in your own words: "With airway obstruction I know something is blocking the air passage between the mouth and lungs." Then rephrase the question: "If there is an obstruction between the mouth and lungs and the patient has been in an auto accident, what are some possible conditions?" By placing the question in a framework that you understand, you will be able to cut through extraneous data and identify the heart of the stem. The answers are the tongue against the pharynx, a crushed larynx, or possible presence of a foreign object.

You can also state the question as a process: "What can block an airway in a trauma patient?" This allows you to follow the process to a logical conclusion (usually the correct answer). *Principle: Rephrase the question in your own words so that it is clear in your mind.* If possible, think of the correct answer before considering the distractors. If you do not know the answer, the following cues to working with distractors may prove helpful.

Principle 4

Distractors are various alternatives chosen to be as close as possible to the right answer. In good test construction, all distractors should be feasible and reasonable and should apply directly to the stem. There should be a commonality in all of the distractors. If one distractor is off base and not plausible, then you can safely assume the person writing the test question ran out of reasonable distractors. *Principle: When analyzing the distractors, isolate what is important in the answer alternatives from what is not important, relative to the question.* In other words, all distractors may be correct but not the right choice for the specific question that is asked. One method of helping you choose the correct answer is to ask yourself whether each possible alternative is true or false in relation to the stem.

> *Example Question:* Parents who abuse their children exhibit all except one of the following characteristics:
>
> A. They have very low impulse control. TRUE
> B. They are socially isolated and lonely people. TRUE
> C. They have realistic expectations of their children. FALSE
> D. Often they were abused as children. TRUE

Asking yourself which distractor is true or false is a shortcut method of answering the question. It forces you to keep looking at the stem. Otherwise, you are trying to judge all of the choices at once. After you have completed the true-false process, remember to go back to the stem and ask yourself if your choice is, in fact, answering the question.

Principle 5

An answer alternative may be correct as it stands by itself, but wrong in terms of what the question is asking. Many, many students fail to recheck the answer with the stem, and they answer the question incorrectly.

An effective strategy in assessing test questions is to judge all four alternative choices against the stem, not against each other. Read the stem, then check Alternative A against the stem, then check Alternative B against the stem, and so on. This process will eliminate choosing an alternative that does not fit with the question. *Principle: After choosing the correct answer alternative and separating it from the distractors, go back to the stem and make sure your choice does, in fact, answer the question.*

Principle 6

If you are answering a test question in which one distractor is considerably different from the others, it is probably not the correct choice. Often, students tend to pick this alternative just because it is different. For example, if the question requires that you select the correct percentage of burn surface area and three of the distractors are in multiples of 9 and one is not, the most likely answer is one of the three alternatives given in a multiple of 9. Sometimes the correct answer will be in direct opposition to the three distractors. In this case, the answer selection will be obvious to you because the other three alternatives will be similar to each other but will not answer the question correctly. *Principle: Look for similarities in two or three of the choices remembering that the purpose of distractors is to divert you from the one right answer.*

Principle 7

The multiple-variable question is one in which each possible answer to the question includes several variables. An effective technique for handling multiple variables is to use the process of elimination. First, study the question and ask yourself what variable fits with this condition, or, after examining the distractors, underline the variable that you know is correct. Now ask yourself what variable is not present with this condition. Again, examine the distractors and cross out those variables which are incorrect. By this process, you probably will have eliminated at least two distractors even without taking the time to consider the other two. *Principle: When a question contains multiple variables as alternative choices, use the elimination-of-variable technique.*

> *Example Question:* To control external bleeding from the forearm, the EMT management includes:
>
> A. Direct pressure, sterile dressing, and lowering of the arm.
> B. Splinting, elevation of arm, and ~~occasional removal of dressing to observe for bleeding~~.
> C. Pressure point, lowering of limb, and sterile dressing.
> D. Elevation of limb, direct pressure, and sterile dressing.

Using the elimination-of-variable technique, first underline the EMT care you know is correct: pressure and sterile dressing. Then cross out the actions you know are wrong: removal of dressing (you know that a dressing is not removed after application because it will disturb blood clots and increase bleeding). Your choices are now between A, C, and D, and you have only to discriminate between elevating or lowering the arm. The answer is D, because elevation of the arm above the heart would reduce the blood flow and thus reduce bleeding.

The Four Basic Question Types

It is important to know that there are different types of questions and, therefore, different types of answers. By recognizing the question type, you can orient your own thinking to the kind of EMT knowledge that you must apply. Furthermore, by recognizing the question type, you may be able to eliminate one or two of the distractors immediately. The four basic question types described in this section are factual, clinical application, quantitative analysis, and clinical judgment.

Factual Questions

The first type of question and the easiest to recognize is a factual one. The question is phrased so that it is asking you for facts or specific EMT knowledge. The distractors will also be factual. This type of question may involve labeling a condition, recalling information, recognizing or defining content.

Example Question: The presence of blood in the chest cavity is:

A. Pericardial tamponade.
B. Pneumothorax.
C. Hemothorax.
D. Subcutaneous emphysema.

The answer is C. Hemothorax is the presence of blood within the chest pleural space outside of the lungs. In order to answer this question correctly, you must know the definitions and associate the correct one with the condition described in the question.

Factual questions also include conceptual issues, that is, dealing with several ideas. For example, a straight factual question might ask you to give the best explanation of congestive heart failure. A factual-conceptual question could ask you to identify which problems a person with congestive heart failure might encounter in his daily living activities. To answer this type of question, you must deal with several ideas or facts that you have learned about this particular condition.

Clinical Application Questions

The second type of question you will find on certification exams is one requiring application in the field. You will solve a problem by using your general EMT knowledge. This type of question will ask you to translate, apply, interpret, demonstrate, or illustrate knowledge or competency in a particular situation. Many EMT certification exam questions fall into this category. Application questions are more "real" because they provide "lifelike" situations. Remember, these exams are attempting to judge you as a safe practitioner. Thus, it is appropriate to present you with specific situations that ask you to apply your EMT knowledge and competency.

> *Example Question:* As an EMT, you realize the danger of administering high-concentration oxygen to a patient with emphysema is:
>
> A. Hypoxia.
> B. Apnea.
> C. Atelectasis.
> D. Dyspnea.

The question demands that you apply basic knowledge of physiology, oxygen therapy, and medical terminology. The answer is B. Oxygen administered in high concentration to the emphysemic patient depresses the normal stimulus to breathe and can cause decreased ventilation to the point of apnea (no breathing).

This type of question demonstrates why you should have a firm understanding of basic anatomy and physiology as well as pathophysiology. It is virtually impossible to keep a great number of random facts in your mind for instant search and retrieval. When you are able to conceptualize facts and put them into an organized format, these facts are more accessible to you. If you understand the way the body works and what can potentially go wrong, you do not have to memorize lists of signs and symptoms. When you are presented with the question, you can figure out the correct response based on your overall knowledge of the body processes. This is basic problem solving that you have learned throughout your EMT education. First, you assess the situation, collect data, and organize it; then you identify the problem and determine the EMT management. This last step involves EMT intervention where you will exercise your clinical judgment, for there are times when you can give high-concentration oxygen and times when you do not. Your clinical judgment should be based on basic knowledge of physiology, pathophysiology, and problem solving rather than attempting to remember a myriad of isolated facts.

Quantitative Analysis Questions

The third type of question you will encounter is a quantitative analysis question. You will be required to separate information into component parts to solve a problem or calculate an answer.

> *Example Question:* An adult male has second-degree burns covering both arms. Using the rule of 9's, what is his category of burn?
>
> A. Minor.
> B. Moderate.
> C. Critical.
> D. None of the above.

The answer is B. After translating the man's burns into a percentage (each arm = 9%, or 2 x 9% = 18%), you can determine that he has moderate burns. Second-degree burns involving 15–25% of the adult body surface are considered moderate.

In this type of question, you completed the analysis by performing a calculation. As with clinical application questions, you must have the basic information upon which to base your analysis. Guessing will be hazardous, so master the EMT knowledge required, such as calculations, rules, and actions of common drugs.

Clinical Judgment Questions

The fourth type of question, and the most discriminating in terms of assessing the individual's ability in emergency situations, is the evaluation question asking for clinical judgment. When you must discriminate between EMT interventions, when you must choose the action you would do first or the one with the highest priority, you are directly demonstrating your level of competence in emergency situations.

This type of question asks you to make a judgment, evaluate, predict, value, select, assess, and finally choose an appropriate action. It is the most sophisticated type of question you will encounter and the one that will require all your knowledge and EMT experience to answer correctly. State and National Registry exams may be oriented more and more toward this type of question because it effectively assesses your level of competency to practice safe EMT care.

To make clear judgments, you must not depend on memorization or recall. You will have to employ the problem-solving process and, as stated earlier, this is the best reason to know pathophysiology along with diseases, signs and symptoms, medical management, and EMT intervention.

Evaluation questions can be divided into two groups, both of which require EMT judgments. The first type of question requires EMT action, and the second, an EMT response. Let us look at an example of a question asking for clinical judgment on an EMT action.

> *Example Question (Action):* Mr. Moreno has been involved in a barroom fight. He has been stabbed once in the right chest wall and once in the left upper arm. You are on the first responding ambulance and have arrived four minutes after the call was received. Upon an initial examination, you find the patient has profuse bleeding from the left arm wound, his chest wound is sucking, and he appears cyanotic and anxious. Your first action would be to:
>
> A. Apply direct pressure to the arm wound.
> B. Administer high-concentration O_2.
> C. Seal the sucking chest wound.
> D. Lay the patient on his left side.

This question is asking for an EMT judgment—the first EMT action under these specific conditions. You must assess the data, identify the problems, identify the **immediate patient need**, and make a judgment about the appropriate EMT intervention. You are now using the problem-solving process.

The answer is C. Seal the sucking chest wound first to prevent any further air entering the chest cavity and allow better ventilation. Subsequently, you may control the bleeding from the arm by use of direct pressure, give him oxygen as his ventilatory abilities are compromised, and proceed with dressing, vital signs, and complete patient exam. You may choose to transport him on his side, but the **right** side would be preferred. Most of the answer alternatives are correct under certain circumstances. However, you are asked to make a judgment about the **most** correct response or first EMT action.

The second type of evaluation question requires an EMT response and usually is based on communication principles. In answering this type of question, you must be especially careful to read the question clearly and understand exactly what it is asking.

Example Question (Response): You are called to a "jumper" and find Mrs. Sarver is depressed and suicidal. She states that she has no reason to live, now that her last child has left home for work in another city. The EMT can best respond to this statement by saying:

A. "I care about you and want you to live."
B. "Your husband is home and he still needs you."
C. "Your daughter cares about you. You said she calls every day and is coming to visit you tomorrow."
D. "Life doesn't look very good to you right now, does it?"

Considering Mrs. Sarver's condition, symptoms, and statement, you are now asked to make a judgment concerning the best EMT response. From your knowledge about communication, you are aware that Responses B and C are not appropriate because they invalidate the patient's feelings. Under some circumstances, Response A could be appropriate, especially if a depressed person feels no one cares about him or her. In this question, however, Response D is correct because Mrs. Sarver's feelings and experience need to be acknowledged and validated, not denied. In order to have selected this response, you had to utilize your EMT knowledge about depressed patients and the communication process, and also make a judgment that applies to this particular situation.

You may encounter an evaluation question that offers you four responses, none of which you would normally choose. The key to answering this type of question is identifying the answer with the greatest therapeutic value.

Example Question: You arrive at the scene of an unknown illness and find a 64-year-old female unconscious and cyanotic on the floor of her kitchen. You are unable to establish an airway and ventilate although you have repositioned her head twice. Your next step is to:

A. Check for pulse.
B. Stop resuscitation attempt.
C. Reposition and attempt another ventilation.
D. Start O_2 with a mask.

The answer, like it or not, is C. The rationale in choosing this response is that the other options do not provide the open airway. Although C is a repeat of actions that have failed already, checking for a pulse, starting O_2, or stopping resuscitation will not improve the patient's airway status.

Test-Taking Strategies

Several test-taking strategies can provide you with useful rules of thumb in answering questions. These strategies are suggested to act as a guide, not an absolute, in choosing the best response for the question.

1. Your first "hunch" is usually correct. Many of us have a first impression, choose an answer, and then, upon reflection, go back and change the answer. A "feeling" that a particular alternative is right has some basis. It is simply that your brain made rapid connections. You came to an immediate conclusion based on your stored knowledge and your experience. The fact that you did not go through the logical steps of arriving at the correct solution does not indicate that your choice is wrong. Research studies have proven that these first impressions are probably correct.

2. Frequently, the most comprehensive answer is the best choice. For example, if two alternatives seem reasonable but one answer includes the other (i.e., it is more detailed, extends the first, or is more comprehensive), then this answer would be the best choice.

3. Eliminate answers that focus on medical knowledge or contain medical management as EMT care. Remember, this is an EMT test and the questions are designed to test EMT competency and safety. It is unlikely that a question would require a medical action for the correct answer; it may, however, offer these actions as distractors.

4. The answer to a question may be found in the following question. You can use this as validation for your choice of alternatives. For example, a condition is described in the first question, and you are asked to label it. If the next question concerns a patient with the same condition, you will be able to validate your answer to the first.

5. You may find several questions grouped in sequence, that is, a group of questions that follow one another and are connected. When this occurs, watch to see that all of your answers fit together and fall within the framework presented.

6. There is no pattern to the answers. The questions are chosen at random, and you may choose the same letter answer for five or more consecutive questions.

7. Beware of answers that contain specific qualifiers, such as "always" and "never." They rarely fit within a logical framework. Remember, however, that some qualifiers are correct, especially in a negative situation. Some situations may be true only when a qualifier is added.

8. It is important that you do not spend several minutes on any one question because your overall time allotment is approximately one minute per question. If you lose time and become immobilized, this will interfere with your cognitive processes for the rest of the test. Leave the time-consuming questions (those that are excessively long or are difficult to comprehend or those that focus on subject matter with which you are unfamiliar) and come back to them after you have completed the test. Remember, if you skip a question, also leave a blank space on the computer sheet or all the succeeding answers will be wrong.

9. Looking at the odds, if you really have no idea of the correct answer, you may choose to leave this question and go on. Blind choices give you only a 25% chance of guessing correctly. You may find the answer contained in later questions.

10. Where "all of the above" or "none of the above" appears as an alternative distractor, it is likely to be the correct answer.

In summary, these strategies are guidelines, not absolutes. Always use your own judgment, knowledge, and EMT experience. These assets will serve you well in passing EMT certification exams. You have the background, education, and knowledge to pass these exams. Let your own creative abilities come through. Be confident that you will pass and, in fact, you will.

Review Guidelines

Most students have only a few weeks between final examinations at EMT school and the state or National Registry examinations. It is very important that the review process be conducted in an efficient manner. The following recommendations illustrate ways that you can achieve maximum results for the amount of review time invested.

Use regularly scheduled periods for study and review. Arrange to study when mentally alert; if you study during periods of mental and physical fatigue, your efficiency is reduced. When studying, use short breaks at relatively frequent intervals. Breaks used as rewards for hard work serve as incentives for continued concentrated effort. Remember, be good to yourself, and when you work hard you deserve a reward.

Analyze your own strengths and weaknesses. Consider your past performance on classroom tests and written applications of factual material. Try to recall the types of questions (factual, judgmental, etc.) that you have been missing. Remember to systematically eliminate your weaknesses. Allow sufficient time for repeated review of those areas that continue to pose problems.

Set priorities on the material that is to be learned or reviewed. Identify the most helpful sections in your notes and review books, and underline or highlight the essential thoughts. Think of examples that illustrate the main points you have studied. Recall examples from your own practical experience or from clinical cases about which you have read. Solidify newly learned material by writing down the main ideas or by explaining the major points to another person.

Test yourself by answering the practice questions in this review book. In addition to studying answers and their rationales, concentrate on understanding the underlying principles and reasons for the answers. Acquire flexibility to answer questions phrased in different ways over the same range of content. Important concepts may be tested repeatedly in the exams, but the questions will be phrased differently.

Become familiar with the examination format. Study the format used for state examinations so you know the different ways in which questions are asked. When answering the questions in this book, set time limits for covering a given unit of questions (approximately one minute per question) to establish the habit of testing under time pressure.

Maximizing Your Testing Effectiveness

The following suggestions will help you to maximize your testing effectiveness. Get a good night's rest. Don't stay up all night learning new materials. Avoid the use of stimulants or depressants, either of which may affect your ability to think clearly during the test. Approach the test with confidence and the determination to do your best. Think positively and concentrate on all you **do** know rather than on what you think you **do not** know.

Consider traveling to the test site several days in advance so that you are sure of your route, parking accommodations, and room location. On the day of the exam, eat a good breakfast. Allow ample time to travel to the testing site, including time to park and to get to the proper room. Choose a location in the testing room where you are least likely to be distracted and where you are away from friends.

During the exam, carefully read the directions for the test to fully understand how to proceed. Review the scoring rules and understand the penalties for incorrect answers. Remember that if you skip too many questions, you may not accumulate enough points to pass the examination. For each test, determine the total number of questions, and estimate how much time you have for each question. Keep track of your progress against your time schedule.

Anxiety—A Potential Problem That You Can Control

Anxiety, the strongest deterrent to successful test taking, interferes with your ability to effectively use your cognitive processes. Anxiety blocks the search and retrieval process so that the knowledge held in your "memory bank" is inaccessible. Fear of the unknown is a major source of anxiety. This fear can be overcome by diligent review which, as you gain mastery over the EMT content, increases your self-confidence. Also important is an understanding of test construction and a strategy for taking tests. The chapter that you have just completed was designed to eliminate many of the unknowns associated with state and National Registry exams and to provide you with test-taking strategies and techniques.

2 Roles and Responsibilities of the EMT

The information contained in Chapter 2 is presented to help you better understand the history of emergency medical services, the role of the EMT as a health care professional, and the EMT's legal accountability.

As a health care professional with a wide range of responsibilities, the EMT must have mastery over a specific set of skills and knowledge. Since it is common to hear such terms as "malfeasance" and "malpractice" used inappropriately, terminology questions are presented to help enlighten the EMT by presenting brief definitions of some commonly used medicolegal terms. You will be required to possess a thorough knowledge of the EMT's duties, standards of care, and consent laws.

1. Emergency Medical Services, as we know it today, was established when the Committee on Trauma and Shock of the National Academy of Science, National Research Council, published the white paper "Accidental Death and Disability: The Neglected Disease of Modern Society" in:

    A. 1964.
    B. 1966.
    C. 1970.
    D. 1973.

2. Called to a pedestrian accident, you find a blind male who was hit by a motorist while crossing the street. His injuries are limited to a closed fracture of the lower leg. During your care for this patient, it is important to:

    A. Lower the head of the stretcher.
    B. Carefully explain all of your actions.
    C. Delay questioning until arrival at the Emergency Department.
    D. Never use the siren while transporting a conscious blind patient.

3. An out-of-state EMT comes upon a person injured in an automobile accident. He must:

    A. Notify the local hospital.
    B. Stay with the patient until adequate care is rendered.
    C. Notify the appropriate police agency, using 911.
    D. Notify the local ambulance service.

4. When parking an ambulance at the scene of an accident, it is advisable to park:

    A. Next to the accident on the shoulder.
    B. In front of the accident.
    C. Next to the accident near the center line.
    D. Behind the accident.

5. An EMT's "standard of care" is judged by comparing his actions to:

    A. The actions of a paramedic (or nurse).
    B. The actions of a similarly trained EMT.
    C. The care rendered in a hospital emergency room.
    D. Optimum care standards.

6. Upon return to your base station, you discover a mistake on your last patient care form. In order to correct your records you should:

   A. Erase the mistake.
   B. Scribble over the mistake so it is not legible and write the correct entry.
   C. Draw a single line through the mistake, then initial and date it.
   D. Tear up the inaccurate report and complete a new one.

7. The formal documentation of certain types of training, privileges, and abilities is:

   A. Licensure.
   B. Certification.
   C. Professional standard.
   D. Standard of care.

8. You have responded to a one-car accident. Lisa Hoffman, the driver of the car, is not seriously injured. She appears to be under great stress and expresses worry about the damage to her car and possible injury to her golden retriever. Your most appropriate response is:

   A. "Everything will be fine."
   B. "You do have insurance, don't you?"
   C. "Yes, I can understand your concerns."
   D. "Don't worry about your car or dog now; your health is more important."

9. Your examination of Lisa reveals normal vital signs, a 2-inch laceration above her left eye, and some bruises on her knees. She also complains about blurred vision, which she states is normally corrected with her glasses (broken in the accident). You should:

   A. Transport to the Emergency Department.
   B. Bandage the laceration and call her family to take her and the dog home.
   C. Ask the police if you should transport.
   D. Secure her health and auto insurance information before transporting.

10. An adult patient is found unconscious. Treatment of this patient will be administered under what type of consent?

    A. Actual consent.

B. Informed consent.
C. Valid consent.
D. Implied consent.

11. Any action outside the scope of practice or standards of care imposed by administrative order, ordinance, or statute is said to create:

    A. Informed consent.
    B. Presumptive negligence.
    C. Immunity.
    D. Professional standards.

12. A family physician has called your service to transport an 80-year-old male whom he believes has suffered a slight stroke. The man is conscious and refuses to be transported. You should:

    A. Transport since the physician diagnosed a stroke.
    B. Return to quarters.
    C. Seek permission to transport from the man's daughter.
    D. Determine the patient's competency and secure written refusal for treatment.

13. Generally, an EMT is required to report certain types of cases encountered including:

    A. Suspected child abuse.
    B. Injuries received during public sporting events.
    C. Drug overdose by an addict.
    D. Injuries received in an industrial accident.

14. The best legal defense for an EMT is to:

    A. Uphold the Good Samaritan laws.
    B. Maintain malpractice insurance.
    C. Skillfully render required care.
    D. Maintain current certification.

15. A 16-year-old married female requests your assistance in giving childbirth. Many states would regard this type of consent as:

    A. Minor's.
    B. Implied.
    C. Actual.
    D. Parental.

16. To perform a medical duty without a patient's consent is:

    A. Nonfeasance.
    B. Misfeasance.
    C. Disfeasance.
    D. Malfeasance.

17. A patient is considered to have withdrawn consent if he or she refuses treatment:

    A. In an instant of pain.
    B. Knowing the consequences of the cessation of treatment.
    C. In anger.
    D. Even when his or her life is threatened.

18. When you arrive at the scene of an accident, a well-dressed female identifies herself as a physician. You should:

    A. Request identification.
    B. Advise the woman that she can provide care only if Medical Control allows her to do so.
    C. Refuse any assistance unless the physician has staff privileges at your base hospital.
    D. Perform and document all of the woman's orders.

19. Proper medical records (prehospital report forms) or charting is essential. Which of the following documentations demonstrates good charting?

    A. "Blood pressure not taken due to burns on extremities."
    B. "The patient is drunk."
    C. "B.P. 120/80, P. normal, R. normal."
    D. "Patient is shocky."

20. You are treating a male patient, approximately 25 years old, who has received an open fracture to the left lower leg. He was hit by a car while crossing the street. He does not speak to you and constantly points to his leg and then his abdomen. You suspect that the patient:

    A. Has a head injury.
    B. Is learning disabled.
    C. Is drunk.
    D. Is a deaf mute.

21. Routine at an accident scene might allow for the:
    A. Assumption of police functions even when police are present.
    B. Questioning of relatives in the presence of the patient.
    C. Use of volunteer help.
    D. Removal of "hot" power lines from wrecked automobiles.

22. You are caring for a victim of a hit-and-run motor vehicle accident. Select the proper action or response in communicating your suspicions that the victim has been drinking.
    A. The prehospital care form should state that the patient "is under the influence of alcohol."
    B. The radio transmission to Medical Control should state the victim's name and your suspicion of alcohol involvement.
    C. Medical Control should be informed that there is a possible presence of ETOH.
    D. The prehospital care form should state that the patient's injuries may be caused in part by his being drunk and that he stepped out in front of the passing vehicle.

23. While working for a volunteer ambulance service, you respond to a small manufacturing plant for a "man down." Upon your arrival you see a second worker stumble to his knees and fall near another person on the ground. As the first arriving EMS unit, your first responsibility on the scene is:
    A. Preservation of the scene.
    B. Evacuation of surrounding buildings.
    C. Personal safety.
    D. Patient care.

Answers with Rationale

1. (B) The white paper report was published in 1966, bringing the delivery of emergency medical care into focus throughout the nation.

2. (B) Like sighted people, the blind are often anxious when presented with an unfamiliar situation. A good line of communication will help alleviate many fears. Use of the siren is probably not justified, but if it is needed, advise the patient before it is used.

3. (B) Once he has started to render care, the EMT must stay with the patient until properly relieved by other health care providers or until care is no longer needed. In most states, the EMT is not legally required to stop if he is not identified as an EMT.

4. (B) The best place to park an ambulance is in front of the accident on the pavement. Parking in front affords you an exit route after loading the patient into the ambulance and good footing while walking. Also, traffic is less obstructed. Remember always to protect yourself as well as the patient.

5. (B) An EMT's actions would be compared to those of a similarly trained EMT providing care under the same conditions and using the same available equipment. Optimum care is desirable but generally considered outside of the standard of care.

6. (C) Medical records are considered legal documents and may be subpoenaed as evidence. Any alteration to a legal document requires that the error be struck out with a single line so that it remains legible and then initialed and dated if changed after the record has been completed. Corrections may also be added to the end of the report or recorded on a supplemental form which must also be signed and dated.

7. (B) Certification is a notice of ability or training completed. Licensure allows you to act. A professional standard generally is a published standard of care. Standard of care is what should or should not be done.

8. (C) Validation of the patient's concerns or feelings is most important. Responding that everything is fine or telling her not to worry closes off

the line of communication between you and Lisa. The question of insurance may make the patient defensive and she may refuse your care.

9. (A) Ms. Hoffman should be transported; possible injuries could include head, neck, knees, or hips. You, the EMT, are the medical person and should not ask the police to make a medical decision. Billing information can be gathered en route. If the dog is injured, law enforcement personnel or a family member may call the Humane Society or take the animal to a veterinary hospital. Again, your primary responsibility is patient care.

10. (D) Implied consent is valid only in a true emergency. An unconscious patient would fall into this category.

11. (B) Violation of local scope of practice or statute will create presumptive negligence. The defendant is presumed guilty until evidence is introduced that would permit a deviation from the legal standard. An example might be an EMTA using a pneumatic counter-pressure device while the local custom allows only an EMT-I to use such a device.

12. (D) Your best action would be to attempt to determine his competency and then get a written refusal of treatment signed by the patient. Although the physician has requested transportation, the patient is in control of himself if found to be competent. The daughter would not be able to give valid consent unless guardianship had been awarded by the court.

13. (A) Most states require persons with knowledge of suspected child abuse to report it either to law enforcement agencies or the State (Children's Services Division, etc.). The U.S. Supreme Court has held that drug addiction is not a crime, but rather an illness. Suspected possession or sale of drugs may need to be reported. EMTs are not required to file accident reports which do not generally involve the police.

14. (C) The best legal defense an EMT can have for suits alleging negligence is the demonstration that care was skillfully rendered. Good Samaritan laws and malpractice insurance do very little to prevent an EMT's being found guilty of gross or wanton negligence. Current certification may be of some value in avoiding presumptive negligence.

15. (C) Many states treat minors as adults for the purpose of consent if they are married, pregnant, or emancipated.

16. (D) Malfeasance is performance of a medical duty without a patient's consent. Misfeasance is failure to perform a duty properly. Nonfeasance is failure to perform the duty.

17. (B) A patient has the right to change his or her mind about treatment, but you should do all you can to inform the patient of the consequences of refusing treatment. Consent of a patient is generally not considered withdrawn in a moment of pain or anger. If the injury or illness is life-threatening, it is an EMT's duty to continue treatment.

18. (A) This situation can be difficult to handle. Request identification of medical licensure. If the person is a physician, contact your Medical Control and encourage the intervening physician to determine who will care for the patient. If the on-scene physician assumes care, he or she must accompany the patient to the receiving facility. The physician should also sign a document transferring patient care responsibility from the EMS system and base hospital to herself or himself. The physician must also sign all orders given to the rescuers on the patient's prehospital care form.

19. (A) Keeping proper medical records includes recording what was not done and why, as well as what was done. In a court of law, any action not recorded on the chart is considered to have not been done. Pulse and respirations records should reflect rate and quality, not an opinion. What seems normal to you may not to someone else. Statements such as "Patient is drunk" or "Patient is shocky" should be avoided. Record the observations that lead you to this conclusion, not the conclusion itself.

20. (D) You may be alerted that an individual is hearing and speech impaired if the person appears alert but fails to respond to sounds, points to the ears and shakes the head, or gestures in a manner that suggests that he or she wants to write. A repeated sequence of body movements or gestures may be an attempt to communicate. This patient may be telling you his abdomen is also injured.

21. (C) Volunteers are often solicited for help at accident scenes. The EMT should not assume police functions unless requested to do so by the

police. Relatives should be questioned at a distance from the patient to avoid the emotional involvement of either the patient or relatives. This will also allow for uninterrupted care of the patient. "Hot" power lines are seldom handled by EMTs because of the associated danger.

22. (C) Medical Control should be informed of the possible presence of ETOH (ethyl alcohol). Do not state that the patient is under the influence of alcohol or use the patient's name on the air. Your medical record should only note the possible presence of alcohol and not describe the patient as drunk or otherwise impaired.

23. (C) Your first responsibility at any scene is to ensure your own safety. More than one rescuer has made either foolish or hasty decisions to save others and fallen victim, becoming of no use to his partner or the patients. Evacuation of neighboring buildings could be implemented by use of your public address system. However, evacuees could inadvertently pass through contaminated environments. Evacuation of the patient to a safer environment can be carried out by properly protected (turnouts, self-contained breathing apparatus, etc.) fire personnel.

3   Personal Safety

Although this chapter is short in length, knowledge of its subject matter is vital to the EMT's physical and mental well-being. Several questions are included to test the reader's knowledge of effective infection prevention and control procedures. There are also questions on personal protective clothing, fire hazards, and entry into confined spaces. Additional personal safety questions are distributed throughout the remainder of the manual.

1. Approximately how many health care workers in the United States are infected with hepatitis B virus each year?

   A. 250.
   B. 500–600.
   C. 2000.
   D. 12,000.

2. Airborne diseases include:

   A. Meningitis.
   B. Human immunodeficiency virus (HIV).
   C. Hepatitis B (HBV).
   D. Hepatitis C (HCV).

3. Select the highest risk exposure for the transmission of bloodborne diseases.

   A. Blood contact with the eyes.
   B. Blood contact with the nose.
   C. Contaminated needle-stick injury.
   D. Blood contact with an open area of the skin.

4. Select the disease for which there is no protective vaccine.

   A. Hepatitis A.
   B. Measles.
   C. Influenza.
   D. Mumps.

5. Select the correct statement regarding infection control requirements.

   A. EMTs are required to receive HBV vaccine.
   B. If an EMT initially declines to receive HBV vaccine, he or she may at any time opt to take it.
   C. HIV or HBV status of an EMT must be reported to his or her employer.
   D. Only needle-stick exposures should be reported to the EMT's employer.

6. Select the most correct statement regarding infection control procedures.

   A. Employers must provide personal protective equipment, such as gloves and eye protection.

B. Prescription eyewear is adequate protection from splash, spray, and splatter exposures.
C. EMTs are personally responsible for the laundering of personal protection clothing and equipment.
D. Between assignments, EMTs may eat and drink in an ambulance.

7. The majority of needle-stick injuries occur when:

    A. Preparing IVs.
    B. Recapping a needle.
    C. Disposing of the used needle.
    D. The needle is left exposed on the patient litter.

8. Treatment following actual or perceived exposure to communicable disease does not include:

    A. Mandatory prophylaxis.
    B. Notification of the chain of command.
    C. Verification of the patient's health status.
    D. Documentation of the incident.

9. Select the most correct statement regarding dehydration.

    A. Fluids high in sugar can slow the body's rate of fluid absorption.
    B. Frequent urination is a sign of dehydration.
    C. Urine that has a deep yellow color is an indication of proper hydration.
    D. Caffeinated fluid is absorbed by the body faster than plain water.

10. Select the correct statement regarding proper layering of clothing.

    A. The inner layer of clothing should be thick to absorb moisture.
    B. Wool is the best inner layer.
    C. The outer layer of clothing should allow for easy venting of body heat.
    D. Cotton is an excellent material to help prevent chilling that may be caused by moisture.

11. Choose the correct term for body temperature that is above normal.

    A. Hypothermia.
    B. Hyperthermia.
    C. Hypovolemia.
    D. Hypoxia.

12. Proper protection of the rescuer dictates that:

    A. Helmets be worn with the chin strap fastened.
    B. Ear plugs be worn only around helicopters and extrication operations.
    C. Leather-palmed gloves be used when handling automobile crash victims.
    D. Lug-type soles be used in snow conditions.

13. Select the correct statement regarding fire conditions.

    A. Damage to the respiratory system can result from breathing air heated above 120°F.
    B. Carbon monoxide combines with the hemoglobin in red blood cells 20 times more rapidly than oxygen.
    C. Hydrogen cyanide is a colorless gas with a musty hay odor.
    D. Carbon dioxide has a strong, pungent odor.

14. Signs of an impending backdraft include:

    A. Air or smoke billowing out of a burning building.
    B. Cool exterior doors and windows when fire is visible beyond.
    C. Dark, heavy smoke coming from the building.
    D. Audible whistling or moaning coming from the burning structure.

15. The risk of fire associated with vehicle crashes is about:

    A. 10%.
    B. 5%.
    C. 1%.
    D. 0.05%.

16. What is the most important rule regarding entry into confined spaces?

    A. An atmosphere that has less than 21% oxygen will not support human life.
    B. Entry should be attempted only after the environment is made safe by ventilation.
    C. You should never enter a confined space unless it has been determined safe for entry.
    D. Entry is performed only to extricate conscious patients.

17. You are called to the scene of a farming accident where a worker has fallen into a liquid manure confinement structure. You should:

    A. Always request fire personnel to effect the rescue.
    B. Request the fire department to cover the material with foam.
    C. Secure a lifeline and use a boat to reach the victim.
    D. Discontinue the use of any electrical devices in the area.

18. What is the leading cause of farm accident fatalities?

    A. Tractor rollover.
    B. Silo suffocation.
    C. Cornpicker entrapment.
    D. Baler entanglement.

Answers with Rationale

1. (D) The Centers for Disease Control estimate that 12,000 health care workers, specifically including emergency medical workers, become infected with HBV each year. Five hundred to 600 will be hospitalized as a result and approximately 250 will die.

2. (A) Meningitis, mumps, rubella, chicken pox, and tuberculosis are airborne diseases spread by droplets of the disease-producing organism being expelled into the air by a productive cough or sneeze. HIV, HBV, and HCV are bloodborne diseases spread by direct contact with the blood or other body substances of an infected person. It has been estimated that nearly 90% of those infected with HIV are unaware of their infected status.

3. (D) The more direct a route of exposure is to the host's blood, the greater the risk of infection. Blood or body fluid contact to the mucous membrane surfaces of the eyes, nose, and mouth is less threatening than a contaminated needle-stick injury.

4. (A) There is no vaccine available for hepatitis A, human immunodeficiency virus, or meningitis. Vaccines do exist for influenza, measles, mumps, and hepatitis B. No vaccines are available for other types of hepatitis. The current OSHA standards covering bloodborne pathogens require employers to offer HBV vaccination free to all employees who will be exposed to blood or other potentially infectious materials as part of their job duties. This requirement includes organizations that use volunteers to provide health care services.

5. (B) OSHA standards allow an EMT to receive HBV vaccine any time he or she is employed in emergency service even if they have previously declined vaccination. HIV and HBV status is confidential and may only be released to an employer if the EMT gives specific written consent. All potentially infectious exposures should be reported to the EMT's employer for proper medical follow up.

6. (A) It is the responsibility of the employer, or agency, to provide and launder all personal protective equipment. Prescription eyewear should be fitted with solid side shields to protect against splash/splat-

ter exposures. OSHA forbids eating and drinking in the ambulance patient-care compartment. Food or beverage may not be consumed in the cab area of the ambulance if the cab is contaminated with visible blood. An EMT may not eat or drink if his or her clothing is visibly contaminated.

7. (B) Most needle-stick injuries in the prehospital setting occur when needles are recapped; this dangerous procedure should be avoided. Used sharps should be properly disposed in an appropriate container without recapping or bending. "Self-capping" and "self-sheathing" needles reduce the potential for needle-stick injury.

8. (A) Although strongly recommended, postexposure prophylaxis is not mandatory. Notification of the chain of command, verification processes to decide if the exposure poses a danger to the EMT's physical or emotional health, appropriate medical treatment, and careful documentation of the incident are considered essential follow-up to an actual or perceived exposure.

9. (A) Fluids high in sugar and caffeine can slow the body's rate of fluid absorption. Frequent urination can indicate adequate hydration. Urine that has a deep yellow color can indicate dehydration.

10. (C) Outer layers of clothing should resist wind and precipitation and have zippers to aid in venting body heat to avoid overheating. The inner layer should be thin and possess the ability to wick moisture away from the skin. Wool and polyester pile are best used for the thermal layer. Cotton tends to absorb moisture.

11. (B) Hyperthermia is the state of the body temperature being above normal. Adequate hydration and wearing proper clothing to vent heat away from the body can help avoid the effects of hyperthermia. Hypothermia is a lower than normal body temperature condition. Hypovolemia is a decreased volume of blood or other body fluids. Hypoxia is a deficiency of oxygen reaching the tissues of the body.

12. (A) Helmets should be worn in any environment where you are subject to encountering falling objects. Chin straps should be fastened because the first falling object may knock the helmet off, leaving the wearer exposed to additional falling objects. Ear protection should be worn in any environment where high noise levels are present. Rubber gloves should

be worn anytime there is a possibility of blood/body fluid exposure. Rubber gloves should be worn inside leather gloves when handling crash victims. Although lug-type boot soles may provide good traction in snow conditions, the soles will become very slippery when caked with mud or snow.

13. (A) Respiratory tract damage can occur when breathing air heated above 120°F. Carbon monoxide, present in every fire, combines with hemoglobin 200 times more rapidly than oxygen. Carbon monoxide poisoning can range from no symptoms to headache, nausea, vomiting, unconsciousness, and death. Hydrogen cyanide has a noticeable almond odor, while phosgene has a musty hay odor. Carbon dioxide is colorless and odorless. Signs of carbon dioxide exposure include increased respirations, dizziness, and sweating.

14. (D) Audible sounds such as moaning or whistling coming from a burning structure may indicate an impending backdraft. Hot exterior doors and windows, grayish-yellow puffs of smoke, and air or smoke forcefully re-entering a burning structure are also signs of an impending backdraft. Proper respiratory equipment, adequate clothing protection, and a water supply should be in place before entering a burning building. Always stand to the side when opening doors or windows.

15. (D) Although fuel and fuel systems of vehicles involved in crashes present a hazard, less than 0.05% of all automobile crashes involve fire. Smoke from vehicular fires contain many toxic by-products dictating the use of full protective gear to reduce the risk to rescue personnel.

16. (C) While this is a fine point, one should never enter a confined space unless it has been determined safe for entry. First, the atmosphere must be tested to determine potential immediate danger to life and health (IDLH) atmosphere; then, the confined space needs to be thoroughly ventilated. If you are not trained in the proper entry techniques, have trained rescue personnel bring the patient to you for treatment. Any atmosphere that has less than 19.5% oxygen must be considered an immediate danger to life and health. Confined spaces also pose a potential for entrapment, electrocution, drowning, burns, falls, and crush injuries.

17. (C) If your EMS unit has self-contained breathing apparatus available, don the gear and secure a lifeline to yourself and effect rescue from a boat. Have the workers activate the internal ventilatory system or portable fans. Do not attempt to walk on the crust formed over the liquid, even if it appears solid.

18. (A) The most common farm accident fatality is a result of tractor rollover. Extrication is often very difficult because of soft soil. Lifting the tractor is preferred to rolling it off the patient. Silo accidents are typically caused by silo gas. When faced with an accident involving farm machinery, contact the local machinery dealer for help with the extrication. Shut engines off prior to attempting extrications from farm machinery.

4 Anatomy, Physiology, and Diagnostic Signs

A proper understanding of anatomy and physiology of the human body forms a strong foundation from which the EMT can develop a firm and rational approach to prehospital patient care. Several questions are devoted to diagnostic signs and symptoms. Without this knowledge, the EMT cannot effectively communicate the patient's condition to the emergency medical control base station or expect to properly care for the patient. Questions on the kinematics of injury are also included in this chapter. This will help the EMT to better evaluate the potential degree of injury patients may have suffered.

Although many instructors downplay the requirement for a good medical vocabulary, it will become apparent to the EMT that the need to understand the oral communications of the Emergency Department staff makes it imperative that one develops such a vocabulary. One rule to keep in mind is "If you're not sure of what a word means, don't use it!"

1. Which anatomic term is used to describe the back surface of the hand?

    A. Distal.
    B. Inferior.
    C. Dorsal.
    D. Sagittal.

2. While standing with your arms at their natural resting position, you rotated your arms so that the palms face forward. What type of movement was demonstrated?

    A. Flexion.
    B. Extension.
    C. Medial rotation.
    D. Lateral rotation.

3. In what position is a person lying flat on his or her back?

    A. Prone.
    B. Supine.
    C. Lateral recumbent.
    D. Semi-Fowler's.

4. Turning the forearm so the palm of the hand faces downward is:

    A. Abduction.
    B. Adduction.
    C. Supination.
    D. Pronation.

5. As the standing patient faces you, the body surface at the front is the:

    A. Inferior.
    B. Anterior.
    C. Posterior.
    D. Superior.

6. The humerus is in what relationship to the elbow?

    A. Distal.
    B. Inferior.
    C. Proximal.
    D. Superior.

7. The great toe is on which aspect of the foot?

   A. Lateral.
   B. Proximal.
   C. Inferior.
   D. Medial.

8. The most posterior portion of the cranium is the:

   A. Occiput.
   B. Parietal area.
   C. Temporal area.
   D. Basal region.

9. The prominent hard bony mass at the base of the skull, just posterior to the tip of the ear lobe, is called:

   A. Mandible.
   B. Temporomandibular joint.
   C. Mastoid process.
   D. Maxilla.

10. Which of the following organs is found in the neck?

    A. Esophagus.
    B. Aorta.
    C. Venae cavae.
    D. Pulmonary arteries.

11. Beginning with the uppermost component, list in order the structures of the airway.

    A. Bronchus, bronchiole, alveoli, trachea.
    B. Alveoli, bronchiole, bronchus, trachea.
    C. Trachea, bronchiole, bronchus, alveoli.
    D. Trachea, bronchus, bronchiole, alveoli.

12. Of the following structures, which one is found in the thorax?

    A. Sternocleidomastoid muscle.
    B. Thyroid cartilage.
    C. Iliac arteries.
    D. Venae cavae.

13. The lining of the chest cavity is called the:

    A. Pleura.
    B. Peritoneum.
    C. Dura mater.
    D. Diaphragm.

14. Which of the following is located at the inferior end of the sternum?

    A. Jugular notch.
    B. Xiphoid process.
    C. Floating ribs.
    D. Angle of Louis.

15. The apex of the heart lies in the left midclavicular line in the region of the:

    A. Third intercostal space.
    B. Fourth intercostal space.
    C. Fifth intercostal space.
    D. Sixth intercostal space.

16. The arch of the aorta passes:

    A. Anterior to the esophagus.
    B. Lateral to the left side of the spine.
    C. Anterior to the trachea.
    D. Between the trachea and esophagus.

17. In the lower right quadrant of the abdomen, you will find the:

    A. Appendix.
    B. Stomach.
    C. Kidneys.
    D. Pancreas.

18. The upper left quadrant of the abdomen contains the:

    A. Gallbladder.
    B. Spleen.
    C. Ascending colon.
    D. Cecum.

19. The upper right quadrant of the abdomen contains the:

    A. Spleen.
    B. Gallbladder.
    C. Appendix.
    D. Cecum.

20. The genitourinary system includes the:

    A. Pancreas.
    B. Liver.
    C. Rectum.
    D. Kidneys.

21. The bladder lies just posterior to the:

    A. Ilium.
    B. Anterior superior iliac spine.
    C. Ischial tuberosity.
    D. Symphysis pubis.

22. The "innominate bone" is made up of three bones fused together. Which bone is not part of the innominate?

    A. Sacrum.
    B. Ilium.
    C. Ischium.
    D. Pubis.

23. The femoral artery is easily palpated. The femoral nerve and femoral vein lie in what relationship to this artery?

    A. Nerve: lateral   vein: medial.
    B. Nerve: medial   vein: lateral.
    C. Nerve: proximal   vein: distal.
    D. Nerve: posterior   vein: anterior.

24. The ridge of bone easily felt under the muscles in the middle of each buttock is the:

    A. Iliac crest.
    B. Ischial tuberosity.
    C. Inguinal ligament.
    D. Greater trochanter.

25. The bony prominence found proximal to the shaft of the femur is the:

    A. Medial femoral condyle.
    B. Greater trochanter.
    C. Lateral femoral condyle.
    D. Inguinal ligament.

26. The peroneal nerve is located just distal to the knee and is found on which surface of the lower leg?

    A. Anterior.
    B. Posterior.
    C. Medial.
    D. Lateral.

27. The ankle bone is termed the:

    A. Calcaneus.
    B. Medial malleolus.
    C. Lateral malleolus.
    D. Talus.

28. A fracture or dislocation of the medial end of the clavicle would involve the:

    A. Humerus.
    B. Sternoclavicular joint.
    C. Acromioclavicular joint.
    D. "Spine" of the scapula.

29. The bony landmark most posterior to the elbow is the:

    A. Lateral condyle.
    B. Medial condyle.
    C. Olecranon process.
    D. Head of the radius.

30. The knee joint is comprised of all of the following except the:

    A. Tibia.
    B. Fibula.
    C. Femoral condyles.
    D. Patella.

31. The fibrous tissue that encloses skeletal muscles is the:

    A. Aponeurosis.
    B. Fascia.
    C. Tendon.
    D. Ligament.

32. Which nerve do you strike when you hit your "funny bone"?

    A. Ulnar.
    B. Median.
    C. Radial.
    D. Brachial.

33. Which of the following arterial pulse points is located on the lateral aspect of the ventral wrist?

    A. Ulnar.
    B. Radial.
    C. Brachial.
    D. Dorsalis pedis.

34. The section of the spinal column considered the lower back is the:

    A. Thoracic vertebrae.
    B. Lumbar vertebrae.
    C. Sacrum vertebrae.
    D. Coccyx vertebrae.

35. Select a voluntary muscle from the following:

    A. Heart.
    B. Diaphragm.
    C. Bladder.
    D. Hamstring.

36. The systolic blood pressure is the level of pressure present during:

    A. Relaxation of the heart.
    B. Contraction of the heart.
    C. Cardiac contusion.
    D. Minimum pressure phase.

37. The artery used for blood pressure readings in the antecubital fossa is the:

    A. Radial.
    B. Brachial.
    C. Carotid.
    D. Dorsalis pedis.

38. From the following choices select the answer that lists the most easily palpated pulse points.

    A. Brachial, carotid, radial.
    B. Brachial, femoral, dorsalis pedis.
    C. Femoral, carotid, ulnar.
    D. Carotid, temporal, tibialis posterior.

39. Which of the following is considered the proper recording of a vital sign?

    A. Pulse: rapid.
    B. Blood pressure: normal.
    C. Temperature: high.
    D. Temperature: 98.6°F (37.0°C).

40. The usual pulse rate for children age 2 to 4 years falls between:

    A. 70 and 90.
    B. 60 and 100.
    C. 80 and 100.
    D. 100 and 120.

41. The normal respiratory rate of an adult at rest is:

    A. 12–20.
    B. 14–18.
    C. 16–20.
    D. 10–22.

42. The normal diastolic pressure in an adult male is between:

    A. 40 and 80 mmHg.
    B. 65 and 90 mmHg.
    C. 10 and 20 mmHg higher than a female.
    D. 90 and 150 mmHg.

43. A stethoscope should be placed in the ears with the earpieces pointing:
    A. Downward.
    B. Upward.
    C. Backward.
    D. Forward.

44. When using a stethoscope, you should:
    A. Use the bell for low-frequency sounds.
    B. Use the bell for high-frequency sounds.
    C. Press the bell firmly on the skin and make at least a 1/4-inch indentation.
    D. Apply slight pressure on the diaphragm to hold it on the skin.

45. A blood pressure taken by palpation is:
    A. Usually higher than that taken by auscultation.
    B. The diastolic pressure.
    C. Performed with a stethoscope.
    D. The systolic pressure.

46. Skin color changes in a person of color can be checked in the:
    A. Mouth.
    B. Axilla.
    C. Ears.
    D. Feet.

47. The level of consciousness (LOC) of an unconscious trauma patient can be checked by:
    A. Slapping the face.
    B. Pinching the shoulder.
    C. Lifting the arm and releasing it.
    D. Observing the Babinski reflex.

48. Vital signs should be taken:
    A. During the primary survey.
    B. After all fractures are immobilized.
    C. During the secondary survey.
    D. During triage.

49. Using the Glascow Coma Scale, how many points would be given for a patient who responds verbally in an incomprehensible manner?

   A. 1.
   B. 2.
   C. 3.
   D. 4.

50. A patient who opens his eyes to voice command but not spontaneously would receive points on the Glascow Coma Scale.

   A. 4.
   B. 3.
   C. 2.
   D. 1.

51. A respiratory rate of 36 and above would get a Champion/Sacco trauma score of:

   A. 4.
   B. 3.
   C. 2.
   D. 1.

52. A systolic blood pressure of 70–89 mmHg receives a Champion/Sacco trauma score of:

   A. 4.
   B. 3.
   C. 2.
   D. 1.

53. A total Glascow Coma Scale score of 9 would be converted to what score for the Champion/Sacco trauma score?

   A. 5.
   B. 4.
   C. 3.
   D. 2.

54. A primary patient survey should include which one of the following activities?

   A. Controlling minor bleeding.

B. Sealing an open chest wound.
C. Soliciting patient medical history.
D. Splinting.

55. During a secondary patient survey, you should:

    A. Determine the state of consciousness.
    B. Begin treating evident shock.
    C. Stabilize flail chest.
    D. Question patient about movement and sensation.

56. During a secondary patient examination, you should:

    A. Control and cover minor bleeding.
    B. Reinsert protruding intestines.
    C. Remove foreign objects.
    D. Examine for an open airway.

57. During a complete secondary survey, what is checked after the chest?

    A. Upper extremities.
    B. Neck.
    C. Lower extremities.
    D. Abdomen.

58. Your patient is unconscious for unknown reasons. You should:

    A. Remove all clothing.
    B. Search for medical alert emblems and cards.
    C. Transport the patient on his or her back.
    D. Not complete a secondary survey.

59. While assessing a patient's respirations, you should:

    A. Remove all clothing from a male's chest.
    B. Place your hand on the patient's abdomen.
    C. Count for six seconds.
    D. Advise the patient of your actions.

60. When you take a blood pressure by auscultation, place the stethoscope over the brachial artery in the antecubital fossa, which lies slightly:

    A. Lateral on the arm.

B. Medial on the arm.
C. Proximal on the arm.
D. Distal on the arm.

61. Select the best location for starting auscultation of lung sounds.

    A. Center of sternum.
    B. Tip of xiphoid.
    C. Mid-clavicular line, on top of the 12th rib.
    D. Mid-clavicular line, just below the clavicle.

62. Abnormally deep breathing is referred to as:

    A. Apnea.
    B. Hyperpnea.
    C. Tachypnea.
    D. Cheyne-Stokes.

63. Fine, crackling lung sounds are:

    A. Rales.
    B. Rhonchi.
    C. Wheezes.
    D. Croup.

64. Continuous, rumbling, vibratory sounds more easily heard during exhalation are called:

    A. Stridor.
    B. Wheezing.
    C. Rhonchi.
    D. Rales.

65. Which of the following conditions lead to a warm or hot skin temperature?

    A. Heat exhaustion.
    B. Heat stroke.
    C. Blood loss.
    D. Nervous stimulation.

66. A bluish skin color is called:

    A. Jaundice.

B. Bilirubin.
C. Plethora.
D. Cyanosis.

67. The failure of pupils to constrict as a light is shone into the eyes could be caused by:

    A. Diplopia.
    B. Eye disease.
    C. Hyperopia.
    D. Myopia.

68. Paralysis that involves one side of the body is:

    A. Paraplegia.
    B. Hemiplegia.
    C. Quadriplegia.
    D. Lateralplegia.

69. The classic, yet seldom seen, skin color or condition that would lead you to suspect carbon monoxide poisoning is:

    A. Pallor.
    B. Cyanosis.
    C. Mottled.
    D. Cherry red.

70. Match the definitions in the first column with the correct medical abbreviation in the two columns on the right.

    Abbreviations:

A.	As needed.	1.	Fx	7.	gtts
B.	Fracture.	2.	Tx	8.	dil
C.	With.	3.	s	9.	b.i.d.
D.	Without.	4.	c	10.	C
E.	Cancer.	5.	CA	11.	p.o.
F.	Traction.	6.	p.r.n.	12.	h.s.

71. Which scenario will produce the most kinetic energy?

    A. A 150-pound person traveling at 30 mph.
    B. A 180-pound person traveling at 25 mph.

C. A 130-pound person traveling at 35 mph.
D. A 100-pound person traveling at 40 mph.

72. Select the correct statement regarding penetrating injuries.

    A. High-velocity weapons such as M-16s produce greater amounts of cavitation than do most handguns.
    B. Female attackers tend to stab with upward thrusts.
    C. Most knife wounds penetrating the abdominal cavity require surgical exploration to repair damage.
    D. An excellent example of a cavitation-type injury is one that results from a shotgun blast.

73. You have been dispatched to the scene of a two-vehicle MVA. A car has been hit broadside on its left by a delivery step van. You would most expect the driver of the passenger car to have suffered a:

    A. Fractured clavicle.
    B. Fractured ankle.
    C. Ruptured spleen.
    D. Ruptured liver.

74. Which injury pattern is associated more often with pediatric rather than adult auto/pedestrian accidents?

    A. Lower leg fractures.
    B. Pelvic fractures.
    C. Knee injuries.
    D. Chest injuries.

75. How long after death will lividity normally be observed in the body?

    A. 10–20 minutes.
    B. 15–30 minutes.
    C. 45–60 minutes.
    D. Only after several hours.

Answers with Rationale

1. **(C)** The back side of the hand is the dorsum, or dorsal side. It might also be considered the posterior side, while the ventral or anterior surface is toward the front of the body. The term sagittal is an imaginary plane passing from front through back, dividing the body into right and left portions.

2. **(D)** Rotation outward or away from the body's midline would be lateral rotation. Medial rotation would be turning toward the body. Flexion is the act of bending. Extension is the term used to bring the body into or toward a straight condition.

3. **(B)** A person lying flat on his or her back is in a supine position. A prone position is lying face down and flat. A semi-sitting position is known as a semi-Fowler's position. Lying on either side would be a lateral recumbent position. A patient face down on his or her right side and chest, left knee and leg drawn up would be in a Sims position.

4. **(D)** Pronation is inward rotation of the arm to face the palms down. Supination is outward rotation. To adduct is to add or to bring closer to the body. To abduct is to take away. (Think of kidnapping.)

5. **(B)** The patient facing you has his or her anterior surface nearest you. Superior would be used in reference to something that is upper, or toward the head. Posterior means situated behind or toward the rear.

6. **(C)** The humerus is closer to the trunk than is the elbow, so the humerus is proximal to the elbow. The ulna is further from the trunk than the humerus, so it is said that the ulna is distal to the humerus. Inferior means toward the feet.

7. **(D)** The great toe lies toward the midline, thus it is medial. The small toe is away from the midline, thus it is lateral.

8. **(A)** The most posterior portion of the cranium is the occiput. The parietal regions are forward or anterior of the occiput, with the temporal regions being most anterior. Basal is not an area of the cranium; it is a type of skull fracture.

9. (C) The mastoid process is just posterior to the tip of the ear lobe. In serious skull fractures involving the base of the skull, ecchymosis may appear in this area some hours after injury.

10. (A) The esophagus is located in the neck. It starts at the retropharynx (back of the throat) and descends to the stomach. The aorta, venae cavae, and pulmonary arteries are found in the chest cavity.

11. (D) Of the choices offered, the trachea is the uppermost airway component. As air is inhaled, it passes through the trachea toward the lungs where the airway splits into the left and right mainstem bronchus. Further into the lungs the airways become progressively smaller (bronchiole) until the inspired air reaches the alveoli (air sacs) where gas exchange occurs between the air and blood.

12. (D) The venae cavae are the large vessels returning deoxygenated blood to the right side of the heart. The iliac arteries are distal to the aorta in the area of the pelvis. The thyroid cartilage is located just inferior to the larynx. The sternocleidomastoid muscles are found in the neck.

13. (A) The pleura lines the chest cavity; the dura mater covers the brain and spinal cord. The diaphragm divides the thorax from the abdomen. The peritoneum lines the abdominal cavity.

14. (B) The inferior (toward the feet) end of the sternum is the xiphoid process. The jugular notch is superior, as is the angle of Louis. The floating ribs are not attached to the sternum.

15. (C) The apex of the heart, contained in the pericardial sac, is at the fifth intercostal space. This space is the nipple line in male patients. This knowledge can be helpful in determining heart action.

16. (B) The arch of the aorta passes lateral to the left side of the spine. The trachea lies anterior to the esophagus, which is just anterior to the spine.

17. (A) The appendix is normally found in the lower right abdominal quadrant. The upper left quadrant contains the stomach. The kidneys and pancreas are found in both upper quadrants.

18. (B) The spleen is located in the upper left abdominal quadrant.

19. (B) The gallbladder is located in the upper right abdominal quadrant. The appendix and cecum are in the lower right.

20. (D) The kidneys, ureter, urethra, bladder, and reproductive organs make up the genitourinary system. The pancreas, liver, and rectum, along with the intestines, gallbladder, stomach, esophagus, mouth, and throat make up the digestive system.

21. (D) The bladder lies behind the symphysis pubis. Injuries to the bladder are often accompanied by fractures of the symphysis pubis and other pelvic bones.

22. (A) While all of the bones listed form the pelvic girdle, the sacrum is not part of the "innominate bone."

23. (A) The femoral nerve lies lateral and the femoral vein lies medial in relationship to the femoral artery. Remembering the simple acronym NAV will help you to remember this anatomical relationship. The greater the depth of injury, the more likely there would be artery and nerve damage.

24. (B) The ischial tuberosity is the bony prominence found underneath the muscles in the center of each buttock. This is an important landmark used in the application of several brands of traction splints.

25. (B) The greater trochanter is located posterolaterally (or proximally) on each femur just below the joint. The condyles are found distal to the thigh.

26. (D) The peroneal nerve is on the lateral aspect of the lower leg just distal to the knee. It is an important nerve to remember when splinting in this area, as inadequate padding could lead to rapid nerve damage and foot drop.

27. (D) The ankle bone is the talus; the calcaneus is the heel bone; the malleoli are the distal ends of the tibia and fibula.

28. (B) Injuries toward the medial or midline of the clavicle would involve the sternoclavicular joint.

29. (C) The olecranon process is the most posterior portion of the elbow and is part of the ulna. The condyles are the distal humeri.

30. (B) The fibula is not part of the knee, as it does not participate in the articulation of the joint.

31. (B) Fascia is the fibrous tissue that encloses skeletal muscles. Aponeurosis sheets attach muscles to muscles. Tendons attach muscles to bones; ligaments attach bone to bone.

32. (A) The ulnar nerve is the one that is struck when you hit your "funny bone." Remember, the olecranon process is the most posterior portion of the ulna.

33. (B) The radial pulse point is located on the thumb or lateral side of the arm. Face palms forward to determine anterior surface during exam. The ulnar artery is on the little finger side.

34. (B) The lumbar vertebrae make up the lower back. The thoracic is the chest cavity, the sacrum is part of the pelvis, and the coccyx is the tailbone.

35. (D) The hamstring is a large voluntary muscle in the thigh. The heart, diaphragm, and bladder are specialized involuntary muscles.

36. (B) The systolic pressure is the level of pressure found during the contraction of the heart. The diastolic represents the relaxed period of the heart or minimum pressure in the arteries.

37. (B) The brachial artery is used for blood pressure readings in the upper arm. The radial artery is found in the lower arm. The carotid arteries are in the neck; the dorsalis pedis in the foot.

38. (A) The carotid, brachial, and radial pulses are most easily palpated in a normal-sized healthy adult. The more distal arteries are more difficult to palpate, especially if the patient has a low blood pressure (hypotension).

39. (D) The temperature recorded in a numerical designation best represents a vital sign. Statements such as "rapid," "normal," and "high" are somewhat subjective, as these terms may be used differently by each examiner. Vital signs should be recorded in an objective manner.

40. (C) The usual pulse rate for children is between 80 and 100. It is slower in adults, usually between 60 and 100. Infant pulse rates are even more rapid than those in children, generally 100–120 beats per minute.

41. (A) The normal respiration rate for adults is generally within the range of 12–20 breaths per minute. Seldom does a resting, healthy respiration rate exceed 20 breaths per minute.

42. (B) The normal diastolic pressure in a male is between 65 and 90 millimeters of mercury. Females usually have systolic and diastolic pressures 8 to 10 mmHg less than males. Male systolic ranges are generally 90 to 150 mmHg.

43. (D) The earpieces should be pointed forward into the ear canal. They should feel comfortable and exclude outside sound.

44. (A) The bell of a stethoscope should be used for low-frequency sounds. The bell should rest on the skin with no more pressure applied to it than is necessary to isolate environmental sounds. Conversely, the diaphragm is used for high-frequency sounds such as blood pressures and should be pressed firmly on the skin.

45. (D) A blood pressure taken by palpation is the systolic pressure reading and may be slightly lower than if taken by auscultation. It is performed by palpating the radial artery while the BP cuff is deflated.

46. (A) Skin color changes in darkly pigmented people can best be observed in the mouth, sclera (white of the eye), or nail beds.

47. (B) Reaction to painful stimuli can help you to determine the patient's LOC. When a low cervical spine injury is suspected, carefully rub the mastoid bone without moving the head to elicit responsiveness. Slapping the face would be contraindicated in a trauma patient because of possible neck injury. Lifting the arm and releasing it could cause further injury unless the arm was protected or padded.

48. (C) Vital signs should be taken after life-threatening problems are corrected (the primary survey activities). This will provide baseline data early in the patient's course of illness or injury.

49. (B) A patient who responds verbally in an incomprehensible manner to questions would receive a score of 2. No response scores a zero. If the patient is oriented a score of 5 is given. A confused patient receives a 4 and inappropriate responses receive a 3.

50. (B) Opening the eyes only to voice command scores a 3. A patient who opens his eyes spontaneously would score a 4. Eye opening only to painful stimuli is a 2. No eye opening receives a score of 1.

51. (C) A respiratory rate of 36 or above would get a Champion/Sacco trauma score of 2. A rate between 10–24/min scores a 4. A rate between 24–35/min scores a 3. A score of 1 is given to a rate of 1–9 breaths per min.

52. (B) A systolic blood pressure between 70–89 mmHg receives a Champion/Sacco trauma score of 3. A 4 is given to a systolic BP 90 mmHg or above. A systolic BP of 50–69 mmHg receives a 2. A score of 1 is awarded to a BP 0–49 mmHg.

53. (C) When the Glascow Coma score is added to the Champion/Sacco trauma score, it is reduced to approximately one third. A coma score of 9 would convert to a 3.

54. (B) Life-threatening problems should be corrected during the primary patient survey. These problems can include open chest wounds, airway and breathing problems, cardiac arrest, coma, and severe bleeding. Minor bleeding, splinting, and medical history can be addressed during the secondary survey and treatment.

55. (D) The patient should be questioned and observed for movement and sensation during the more complete secondary survey. The patient's state of consciousness (yes or no) should be determined during the initial survey in order to determine the need for protection of the airway. Obvious shock should be addressed by elevation of the legs during primary survey. Flail chests must also be immobilized very early on.

56. (A) Control and cover minor bleeding during the secondary exam. Protruding intestines are never reinserted in the field. Foreign objects are seldom, if ever, removed in the field. The airway should have been initially checked during primary exam.

57. (D) The abdomen is typically examined after the chest. A good secondary exam should always be systematic, starting at the head and working down the body to the feet.

58. (B) It is always a good practice to search for medical alert cards, bracelets, and necklaces for clues to underlying medical conditions that could assist in diagnosis or treatment.

59. (B) A patient's respirations should be assessed by placing your hand on the patient's abdomen. Clothing need not be removed for this procedure. Respirations should be counted for one minute. Do not advise the patient of your actions, as he or she may alter the breathing pattern, rate, or quality.

60. (B) The brachial artery is located slightly toward the midline of the arm and is most easily auscultated with the stethoscope placed over it.

61. (D) Auscultation of the lungs should be done first at a point just below the mid-clavicle, then just below the nipple and about 2 inches laterally, and finally at a point between the 8th and 9th ribs on the posterior thorax.

62. (B) Abnormally deep breathing is hyperpnea. Apnea is absence of breathing. Tachypnea is rapid breathing. Cheyne-Stokes breathing is an irregular or cyclic type of respiration typified by rapid, deep breaths decreasing to a 10- to 20-second period of apnea.

63. (A) Rales are fine, crackling lung sounds much like the sound of strands of hair being rubbed together. Rhonchi are harsher sounds caused by fluid collections in the larger airways. Wheezes are high-pitched sounds heard while air flows through narrowed airways. Croup is a disease typified by noisy, progressively more difficult breathing.

64. (C) Rhonchi are continuous, rumbling, vibratory sounds more easily heard during exhalation. Rales are fine, crackling sounds heard during inspiration and do not clear on coughing as rhonchi. A high-pitched or whistlelike noise found during exhalation is called wheezing.

65. (B) Fever and heat stroke result in the skin feeling hot to the examiner's touch. Heat exhaustion, blood loss, and nervous stimulation present cool, wet (clammy) skin.

66. (D) Cyanosis is a bluish skin color that results from poor oxygenation of the blood. Jaundice is a yellow skin color. Bilirubin is a reddish-yellow pigment deposited in the skin. Plethora is a condition of overfullness of blood vessels, often found in severe hypertension (high blood pressure).

67. (B) Eye diseases can cause failure of the pupils to constrict. Diplopia is double vision. Myopia is nearsightedness and hyperopia is farsightedness.

68. (B) Hemi (meaning half) plegia involves one side of the body. Para (beside) plegia involves both legs. Quadri (four) plegia affects all four limbs.

69. (D) Although seldom seen, the skin of a patient experiencing carbon monoxide poisoning may be cherry red. Pallor is a whitish coloration. Cyanosis is blue skin color. Mottling is a condition marked by discolored areas.

70. As needed (p.r.n.); fracture (Fx); with (c); without (s); cancer (CA); traction (Tx); drops (gtts); dilute (dil); two times per day (b.i.d.); centigrade (C); by mouth (p.o.); hour of sleep or bed time (h.s.).

71. (D) The formula for kinetic energy is equal to one-half of the mass times the velocity squared. The 100-pound person traveling at 40 mph would develop the most KE at 80,000 units of energy. The key to remember in trauma evaluation is the velocity (speed) involved since it is squared. The greater the speeds involved the greater your index of suspicion should be with regard to injuries.

72. (A) High-velocity weapons produce greater amounts of cavitation (cone of destruction) than do most handguns. Shotguns produce fragmentation-type injury patterns. Most female attackers tend to stab in a downward fashion. Only about 30 percent of all knife wounds to the abdomen require surgical exploration to repair damaged organs.

73. (C) Occupants of vehicles involved in a lateral or side impact collision usually have more serious injuries to the side closest to the exterior of the car. Three major areas of injury in this type of crash are to the chest wall, pelvis, and head/neck. A driver's side impact would more likely injure the spleen while a similar crash on the right side would more likely injure a passenger's liver.

74. (D) A child pedestrian will often face forward when about to be involved in a collision while an adult, to protect his or her body, will turn to the side. The child, being shorter, will often suffer thoracic injuries when the hood of the car impacts the chest. Adults will suffer lower leg fractures since the tibia and fibula are often struck by the car's bumper. Knee injuries are experienced by adults as well. Both child and adult are subject to pelvic injury in an auto/pedestrian accident.

75. (B) Dependent lividity will normally occur 15–30 minutes after death and is caused by blood settling in the lower parts of the body. Rigor mortis usually occurs only several hours after death. Rigor mortis is noted as resistance when one attempts to straighten a flexed extremity.

5 Respiratory and Circulatory Systems

This chapter is devoted to testing your knowledge concerning the respiratory and circulatory systems. Many questions on these subjects will appear on your certification exams. It is not uncommon for testing agencies to allocate up to 30% of their written exams to these topics.

The EMT must know the causes of respiratory arrest and how to react quickly to restore the patient's breathing. Cardiopulmonary resuscitation is probably the most important skill for the Basic EMT. The Emergency Cardiac Care information presented in this chapter has been updated to incorporate the new 1992 CPR guidelines adopted by the American Heart Association. Understanding the proper sequence of activities and the rationale behind these sequences will greatly help you master resuscitation skills. Basic principles of defibrillation, including ECG recognition of ventricular fibrillation and nonventricular fibrillation rhythms, are presented in this chapter. The use of manual, automatic, and semi-automatic defibrillators is also reviewed.

Several questions are devoted to the use of suction devices and oxygen administration. Although this area is difficult to test, proper suctioning and oxygen administration is essential knowledge for the EMT.

1. The air we breathe usually contains what percentage of oxygen?

    A. 20%.
    B. 30%.
    C. 70%.
    D. 79%.

2. The exchange of waste products for oxygen occurs in the:

    A. Arteries.
    B. Venules.
    C. Capillaries.
    D. Veins.

3. The leaf-shaped valve that allows gases to pass into the lungs and closes when food or liquid is present is called the:

    A. Esophagus.
    B. Larynx.
    C. Epiglottis.
    D. Pharynx.

4. What prevents the trachea from collapsing during respiration?

    A. Cartilaginous rings.
    B. Pulmonary ligaments.
    C. Positive pressure in the chest upon inhalation.
    D. Negative pressure in the chest upon inhalation.

5. During inspiration, the diaphragm _____ and the rib muscles _____.

    A. Contracts—contract.
    B. Relaxes—contract.
    C. Contracts—relax.
    D. Relaxes—relax.

6. The major stimulus for respiration is normally the arterial blood level of :

    A. Carbon monoxide.
    B. Carbon dioxide.
    C. Nitrogen.
    D. Oxygen.

7. The connection between arterioles and venules is the:

    A. Alveoli.
    B. Artery.
    C. Vein.
    D. Capillary.

8. The smooth, slippery tissue covering the lungs is called the:

    A. Visceral pleura.
    B. Parietal pleura.
    C. Pleural space.
    D. Mediastinum.

9. The space between the lungs is called the:

    A. Mediastinum.
    B. Sternal notch.
    C. Bisternal space.
    D. Hemithorax.

10. Select the organs found in the mediastinum:

    A. Kidneys, lungs, esophagus.
    B. Lungs, trachea, heart.
    C. Aorta, trachea, pancreas.
    D. Trachea, heart, esophagus.

11. Which of the following is considered to be in the upper airway?

    A. Larynx.
    B. Trachea.
    C. Bronchus.
    D. Nasopharynx.

12. The chemical process by which life-maintaining energy is extracted from food is:

    A. Catabolism.
    B. Metabolism.
    C. Epidemiology.
    D. Etiology.

13. The sticky fluid found in the cardiovascular system is the:

    A. Plasma.
    B. Leukocytes.
    C. Erythrocytes.
    D. Platelets.

14. The wall that divides the heart in two is called the:

    A. Atrium.
    B. Ventricle.
    C. Septum.
    D. Mediastinum.

15. The valves between the atria and ventricles are closed. The valves to the arteries are open. Blood will now flow into the:

    A. Right ventricle.
    B. Left ventricle.
    C. Pulmonary artery.
    D. Right and left ventricles.

16. Blood pumped from the right side of the heart travels through the:

    A. Pulmonary vein.
    B. Pulmonary artery.
    C. Aorta.
    D. Venae cavae.

17. The nervous system that continually adjusts the diameter of the blood vessels is the:

    A. Central nervous system.
    B. Reflex.
    C. Voluntary.
    D. Autonomic.

18. The air we exhale usually contains what percentage of oxygen?

    A. 10%.
    B. 16%.
    C. 20%.
    D. 70%.

19. The amount of air usually exhaled during respiration is called the:

    A. Residual volume.
    B. Tidal volume.
    C. Total lung capacity.
    D. Vital capacity.

20. When the brain is deprived of oxygen, brain death usually begins within:

    A. Two to four minutes.
    B. Two minutes.
    C. Six to ten minutes.
    D. Four to six minutes.

21. A patient who is unable to breathe comfortably except when sitting or standing is said to be suffering from:

    A. Orthopnea.
    B. Apnea.
    C. Hypoxia.
    D. Dyspnea.

22. Of the following conditions, which would lead to brain death most rapidly?

    A. Airway obstruction.
    B. Pulmonary arrest.
    C. Angina pectoris.
    D. Cardiac arrest.

23. CPR may be discontinued when:

    A. You are instructed to do so by the police.
    B. You are instructed to do so by a physician.
    C. Your unit receives another call.
    D. The patient becomes deeply cyanotic.

24. Unconsciousness can be established by observing a patient's response to:

    A. Verbal stimuli.
    B. Pupillary reaction to light.

C. Pinching the lobe of the ear.
D. Opening the airway.

25. Rolling an unconscious patient from a face-down position to a recovery position can be best accomplished by:

    A. Bringing the patient's nearer arm above his or her head.
    B. Rapidly pulling up on the patient's belt loops and shoulder.
    C. Pushing the patient's torso away from you.
    D. Lifting the patient away from you.

26. A partial airway obstruction can be identified by all of the following except:

    A. Retraction of the intercostal spaces.
    B. Retraction of the supraclavicular spaces.
    C. Snoring sounds.
    D. Absence of respiratory effort.

27. An unconscious patient's obstructed airway may first be cleared by performing any of the following except:

    A. Forceful mouth-to-mouth ventilation.
    B. Head tilt.
    C. Head tilt–chin lift.
    D. Jaw thrust.

28. The best maneuver for opening an airway in a patient with a suspected neck injury is the:

    A. Head tilt.
    B. Head tilt–chin lift.
    C. Head tilt–neck lift.
    D. Jaw thrust maneuver.

29. The tongue typically blocks an unconscious patient's airway when the neck is:

    A. In flexion.
    B. In hyperextension.
    C. In neutral position.
    D. Extremely large.

30. How many times per minute should artificial ventilation be performed?

    A. 12 times in an adult.
    B. 20 times in an adult.
    C. 8 times in a child.
    D. 14 times in an infant.

31. The period of time allowed for checking unresponsiveness in a patient who appears to be unconscious should be:

    A. Less than four seconds.
    B. Four to ten seconds.
    C. Five to eight seconds.
    D. Ten to twelve seconds.

32. After the airway has been opened, you should:

    A. Ventilate two times.
    B. Palpate the pulse.
    C. Ventilate four times.
    D. Observe three to five seconds for respiration.

33. Appropriate action during your initial ventilatory efforts for a pulmonary arrest patient is to:

    A. Give four full breaths.
    B. Staircase the initial ventilations.
    C. Open the airway for inhalation only.
    D. Observe the chest rise and fall.

34. A patient with a laryngectomy requires:

    A. Head tilt maneuver.
    B. Blowing directly into the tube in the stoma.
    C. Oral suctioning.
    D. Sealing the nose and mouth during exhalation.

35. Which statement about relieving severe gastric distention is correct?

    A. The patient's head and shoulders should remain flat.
    B. A suction device should be ready.

C. The flat of your hand should push on the patient's umbilicus.
D. Severe gastric distention should not be relieved because of the danger of aspiration.

36. The correct hand placement for the Heimlich maneuver is:

    A. On top of the umbilicus.
    B. Between the umbilicus and pelvis.
    C. Between the xiphoid and angle of Louis.
    D. Between the xiphoid and umbilicus.

37. The use of excessive pressure while checking the carotid pulse may cause:

    A. Increased intracranial pressures.
    B. Airway obstruction.
    C. Marked cardiac slowing.
    D. Blood clots.

38. In dealing with an unconscious patient, the hand not being used to check the carotid artery should:

    A. Pinch the nostrils.
    B. Be behind the neck.
    C. Be on the chest.
    D. Maintain head tilt.

39. Your unconscious patient is making snoring sounds and has a pulse of 80. You should:

    A. Start compressions.
    B. Ventilate every five seconds.
    C. Pinch the nostrils closed.
    D. Reposition the head and neck.

40. What is the most common cause of airway obstruction?

    A. Trauma.
    B. Inhaled foreign bodies.
    C. The tongue.
    D. Drowning.

41. What single physiological condition differentiates between clinical and biological death?

    A. Absence of pulse.
    B. Absence of respiration.
    C. Irreversible brain damage.
    D. Unconsciousness.

42. When performing artificial ventilation on an infant, you should:

    A. Use ventilations of 1–1 1/2 seconds each.
    B. Hyperextend the infant's neck.
    C. Ventilate at the same rate as for an adult.
    D. Seal the mouth and pinch the nose.

43. The period of time needed to establish pulselessness in a nonbreathing adult is:

    A. Less than five seconds.
    B. Five to ten seconds.
    C. Ten seconds or more.
    D. Four to eight seconds.

44. The method or maneuver that provides the greatest opening of an airway in an adult is:

    A. Head tilt.
    B. Head tilt–chin lift.
    C. Head tilt–neck lift.
    D. Head neutral–neck lift.

45. You find an unconscious patient, establish unresponsiveness, open the airway, and attempt to ventilate but are unable to do so. Your next action is to:

    A. Apply chest thrusts.
    B. Apply abdominal thrusts.
    C. Apply the finger sweep.
    D. Reposition the head.

46. You are still unable to ventilate the patient after your action in Question 45. Your next action is to:

    A. Apply abdominal thrusts.

B. Apply four chest thrusts.
C. Apply the finger sweep.
D. Reposition the head.

47. You are still unable to ventilate after your actions in Questions 45 and 46. Your next significant action is to:

    A. Apply chest thrusts.
    B. Apply abdominal thrusts.
    C. Apply the finger sweep.
    D. Reposition the head.

48. The proper depth of cardiac chest compressions for an adult is:

    A. 1" to 1½".
    B. 1½" to 2".
    C. 1" to 2".
    D. ¾" to 1½".

49. What percentage of time should be devoted to the downstroke on the compression phase of CPR?

    A. 30%.
    B. 45%.
    C. 50%.
    D. 70%.

50. Two EMTs are performing proper CPR on an adult. Their ratio of compression to ventilation is:

    A. 15:2.
    B. 5:2.
    C. 3:1.
    D. 5:1.

51. How many compressions per minute should be maintained during two-person CPR for an adult patient?

    A. 60.
    B. 70.
    C. 80.
    D. 120.

52. When a second EMT (Bob Guy) joins you in providing CPR, the first activity for you is to:

    A. Check the victim for a spontaneous pulse.
    B. Instruct Bob to check for an artificial pulse.
    C. Give one breath.
    D. Complete your series of compressions.

53. The next activity for you is to:

    A. Check the victim for a spontaneous pulse.
    B. Instruct Bob to check for an artificial pulse.
    C. Give one breath.
    D. Complete your series of compressions.

54. After completion of your activities in Questions 52 and 53, you should next:

    A. Check the victim for a spontaneous pulse.
    B. Check the victim for an artificial pulse.
    C. Give one breath.
    D. Start compressions immediately.

55. After you have completed the activities in Questions 52, 53, and 54, Bob Guy (the second EMT) should:

    A. Give one breath every 5th compression.
    B. Assess your CPR adequacy.
    C. Resume compressions at a rate of 80–100 per minute.
    D. Interpose ventilations during the downstroke of the compressions.

56. When performing adult CPR alone, you should:

    A. Use 15:2 ratio.
    B. Use 5:1 ratio.
    C. Compress at a rate of 60 per minute.
    D. Allow total exhalation after each breath.

57. If you need to interrupt CPR, you should:

    A. Never interrupt CPR for more than 5 seconds.
    B. Interrupt CPR for the time it takes to transport.

C. Never interrupt CPR for more than 30 seconds.
D. Interrupt CPR only when you are tired.

58. A correct statement about infants and children is:

    A. An infant responds to CPR more readily than a child.
    B. Children most often suffer pulmonary arrest.
    C. The majority of cardiopulmonary arrests in infants and children begin with cardiac arrest.
    D. Airway infection does not lead to cardiac arrest in children.

59. When opening the airway of a child, you should:

    A. Not use the head tilt–chin lift method.
    B. Keep the mouth open if the chin lift is used.
    C. Use pressure on the soft tissue under the jaw to help push the chin up.
    D. Open only the airway if the child is cyanotic.

60. When performing mouth-to-mouth ventilation on an infant, you should ventilate:

    A. 12 times per minute.
    B. 15 times per minute.
    C. 18 times per minute.
    D. 20 times per minute.

61. You respond to a frightened mother's call and find a 3-year-old boy in obvious respiratory distress. You open the airway with the chin lift method but are unable to ventilate. The mother states that the child has been ill with a fever for several days. He has had a barklike cough that seems to become weaker. In your best judgment, what should you do for the child?

    A. Transport him immediately.
    B. Attempt four back blows.
    C. Attempt four chest thrusts.
    D. Attempt four abdominal thrusts.

62. Proper care for an infant with an airway obstruction should include:

    A. Hyperextension of the neck.

B. Four back blows before chest thrusts.
C. Blind finger sweeps.
D. Four abdominal thrusts before back blows.

63. The best place to check the pulse of an infant in pulmonary arrest is the:

    A. Carotid artery.
    B. Precordium.
    C. Radial artery.
    D. Brachial artery.

64. After checking the pulse of the infant, you decide to start chest compressions. You should place your two fingers on the:

    A. Upper half of the sternum.
    B. Middle of the sternum.
    C. Sternum one finger above the xiphoid.
    D. Sternum one finger below nipple line.

65. The proper depth of compression for an infant is:

    A. 1" to $1\frac{1}{2}$".
    B. $\frac{1}{2}$" to 1".
    C. $1\frac{1}{2}$" to 2".
    D. 1" to $1\frac{3}{4}$".

66. What is the proper compression rate for infant CPR?

    A. 70.
    B. 80.
    C. 90.
    D. 100.

67. What compression/ventilation ratio should you use while performing one-person CPR on a 6-year-old child?

    A. 15:2.
    B. 5:1.
    C. 15:1.
    D. 5:2.

68. Alone, you find a person in cardiopulmonary arrest. In your judgment, when should you telephone for help?

   A. After the first minute of CPR.
   B. After the patient turns pink.
   C. Before you start CPR.
   D. When you get tired.

69. Properly performed CPR can produce systolic blood pressure peaks of about:

   A. 40 mmHg.
   B. 80 mmHg.
   C. 100 mmHg.
   D. 140 mmHg.

70. The count "One, two, three, four, five, breathe" should be used for:

   A. Infant CPR.
   B. Child CPR.
   C. One-person adult CPR.
   D. Two-person adult CPR.

71. You have just started chest compressions on an adult male. You hear a snapping sound and suspect that you have fractured a rib. Your next action is to:

   A. Reassess your hand position.
   B. Stop compressions.
   C. Compress 1" to 1½".
   D. Rest your fingers over the suspected fracture to keep the rib from breaking the skin.

72. Which of the following is a correct statement about the carotid pulse?

   A. It should always be checked after the first minute of CPR.
   B. It is seldom palpable during external chest compressions.
   C. It can be felt during the diastolic phase of cardiac output.
   D. It is not as good an indicator of circulation as the femoral pulse.

73. The volume of air you give during artificial ventilation is determined by the:

   A. Increased resistance of the lungs.

B. Chest rise.
C. Reduced compliance of the lungs.
D. Ability to blow forcefully for several minutes.

74. To relieve gastric distention in an infant or child, you should:

    A. Compress the patient's chest.
    B. Apply four jabs over the umbilicus.
    C. Hold the patient by the feet and turn him or her upside down.
    D. Turn the entire body on its side.

75. What percentage of oxygen would you expect a patient to receive when using a pocket mask with supplemental O_2 flowing at 10 L/min?

    A. 16%.
    B. 21%.
    C. 32%.
    D. 50%.

76. When using a pocket mask as an adjunct for artificial ventilation, you should:

    A. Use the head tilt–neck lift method.
    B. Maintain a seal on the mouth and nose.
    C. Not be concerned with air leaking during your ventilation of the patient.
    D. Not remove your mouth from the mask at any time.

77. Oropharyngeal (OP) airways may be inserted in a patient when he or she is:

    A. Stuporous.
    B. Gagging.
    C. Unconscious.
    D. Conscious.

78. The insertion of an oropharyngeal airway should be done:

    A. With a dry airway.
    B. Only with the use of a tongue blade.
    C. With the neck in flexion.
    D. With a rotating movement during insertion.

79. What landmarks are used to determine the proper length of nasopharyngeal airway?

    A. Earlobe to nose.
    B. Lips to angle of the jaw.
    C. Nose to angle of the jaw.
    D. Chin to nose.

80. All bag-valve-mask systems should use:

    A. Pop-off valves.
    B. Transparent plastic face masks.
    C. Standard 12/18 mm fittings.
    D. Sponge rubber inside the bag.

81. Suction equipment used during resuscitation should:

    A. Provide 200 mmHg of vacuum.
    B. Use small-bore tubing.
    C. Have metal pharyngeal suction tips.
    D. Have a supply of water available.

82. At the scene of a motor vehicle accident (MVA), you examine the pharynx of a patient and discover blood and other secretions. As you suction this patient, you should:

    A. Insert the suction tip at the base of the tongue.
    B. Apply suction while inserting the tip.
    C. Continually suction until all the secretions are removed.
    D. Apply suction only after the tip is in place.

83. Frothy sputum seen at the mouth could indicate:

    A. Lung contusion.
    B. Head injury.
    C. Infectious hepatitis.
    D. Ketoacidosis.

84. A patient in early stages of hypoxia will exhibit:

    A. Bradycardia.
    B. Tachycardia.
    C. Cyanosis.
    D. Drowsiness.

85. For some COLD patients, use of short-term supplemental oxygen can cause:

   A. Burning.
   B. Decreased CO_2 exhalation.
   C. Toxicity.
   D. Decreased ventilatory drive.

86. Medical gas is generally delivered to a patient at a pressure of:

   A. 2000–2200 psi.
   B. 700 psi.
   C. 50–100 psi.
   D. 40–70 psi.

87. The best guideline regarding the use and handling of oxygen equipment is:

   A. Never fully open the valve without having the regulator attached.
   B. Grease all fittings once a month.
   C. Never use a high-pressure cylinder without an O-ring or washer attached.
   D. Always face the regulator when turning on a tank to observe the needle rise.

88. The "safe residual" level in medical oxygen cylinders is:

   A. 15 liters.
   B. 30 liters.
   C. 200 psi.
   D. 500 psi.

89. You have decided to deliver oxygen to a patient using a nasal cannula. You should:

   A. Expect an oxygen-concentration range of between 25% and 35%.
   B. Determine if the patient can breathe through his or her nose.
   C. Choose a flow rate between 4 and 6 L/min.
   D. Not concern yourself with humidification.

90. A simple face-mask oxygen-delivery system will:

   A. Not need humidification.
   B. Deliver concentrations of oxygen between 30% and 50%.

C. Use a flow rate of 6–10 L/min.
D. Be adequate for use during CPR.

91. The mask and bag (also called nonrebreathing mask) system can:

    A. Be preset at 8 L/min flow.
    B. Deliver 90% O_2 concentrations.
    C. Not be used with a humidification device.
    D. Only be used effectively on adults.

92. Of the following statements about venturi mask systems, which is the most correct?

    A. Humidification is never used.
    B. The system delivers fairly accurate concentrations of O_2.
    C. This system is the most frequently used by EMTs for conscious patients.
    D. O_2 concentration level is affected by changes of rate or depth of respirations.

93. You are performing one-person CPR on a 9-month-old infant. Choose the statement that best fits this situation.

    A. The appropriate size bag-valve-mask device will contain 500–700 cc.
    B. Using the reservoir accessory on the bag, you can deliver a 60% concentration of O_2.
    C. This bag-valve-mask should be equipped with an overpressure pop-off valve.
    D. The bag-valve-mask device is of little value in the situation.

94. When suctioning a patient, the catheter should be inserted:

    A. The distance from the mouth to the lobe of the ear.
    B. As far as possible.
    C. Until gagging occurs.
    D. Only in the mouth.

95. In choosing the proper size of oropharyngeal airway, you should:

    A. Measure from the tip of the lobe of the ear to the corner of the mouth.
    B. Pick a diameter that is half that of the open mouth.

C. Use the longest length you can get behind the tongue.
D. Measure from the tip of the larynx to the corner of the mouth.

96. Nasal cannulas or prongs are frequently preferred for use by EMTs because:

   A. People breathe through their noses.
   B. The patient can talk and not feel smothered.
   C. Prongs are more effective than face masks.
   D. Cannulas do not require humidification.

97. Injuries crushing the larynx or trachea are commonly seen in motor vehicle accidents involving the steering wheel. Proper care for such an injury includes:

   A. Positive-pressure ventilation.
   B. Encouraging the patient to breathe more rapidly.
   C. Hyperflexion of the neck unless cervical spine injuries are suspected.
   D. Encouraging the patient to breathe slowly and administering O_2.

98. If an oropharyngeal airway is too short, you should expect:

   A. Laryngeal spasms.
   B. Vomiting.
   C. Gag reflex action.
   D. Airway occlusion.

99. After the use of humidified oxygen on a patient, you should:

   A. Add more water to the humidifier.
   B. Sterilize the humidifier and change the water.
   C. Sterilize and change water once a week.
   D. Change the water every eight hours.

100. Several concerns arise when moving a patient from the scene of a cardiac arrest into the back of the ambulance while CPR is being performed. Select the proper action.

   A. When moving a patient upstairs, the head of the cot should go up first.
   B. When moving a patient down a flight of stairs, the head of the cot should go first.

C. When lifting a patient onto the cot, grab him or her by the shoulders and lift the head higher than the feet.
D. When lifting the cot into the ambulance, lift from the side rails instead of the frame.

101. Which of the following would you consider to be the most important factor in a successful resuscitation attempt?

    A. CPR is begun within 4–6 minutes of the patient's collapse.
    B. A defibrillator is available within 15–20 minutes of collapse.
    C. Full advanced life support treatment is available to the patient within 20–25 minutes of collapse.
    D. The patient must be found in ventricular fibrillation in order for EMT-Ds to provide care.

102. Select the response that identifies the normal conduction pathway of electrical impulses traveling through the heart.

    A. SA node, bundle of His, AV junction, bundle branches.
    B. AV junction, bundle of His, SA node, bundle branches.
    C. Bundle of His, SA node, AV node, bundle branches.
    D. SA node, AV junction, bundle of His, bundle branches.

103. Which of the following ECG tracings identifies the contraction of the ventricles?

    A. P-wave.
    B. QRS complex.
    C. T-wave.
    D. PR interval.

104. You respond to a call at an adult foster home where a care provider tells you that an elderly patient fainted. The ECG shown below depicts a/an:

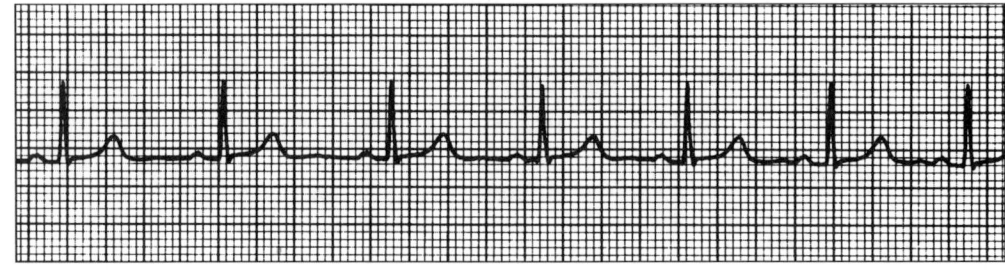

A. Ventricular tachycardia.
B. Heart rate of over 120.
C. Irregular rhythm.
D. Normal sinus rhythm.

105. Select the correct statement regarding the electrical system of the heart.

    A. Ventricular tachycardia often lasts more than three minutes.
    B. A patient in ventricular tachycardia will not have a palpable pulse.
    C. No peripheral pulses can be felt in a patient in ventricular fibrillation.
    D. Asystole often precedes ventricular fibrillation.

106. The following ECG is representative of:

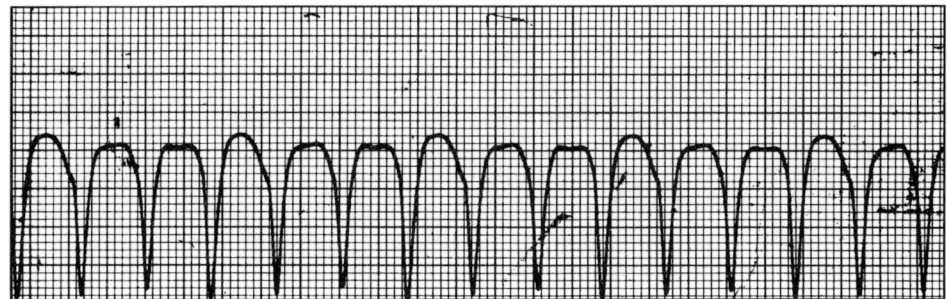

    A. Ventricular tachycardia.
    B. Ventricular fibrillation.
    C. Asystole.
    D. Normal sinus rhythm.

107. The following ECG is representative of:

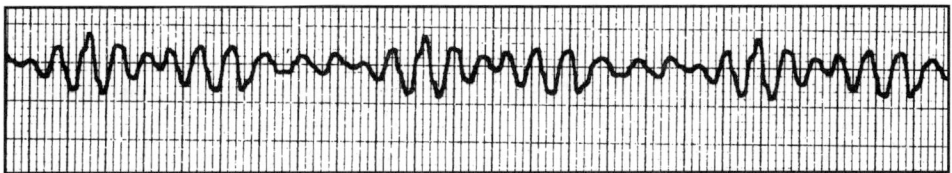

    A. Ventricular tachycardia.
    B. Ventricular fibrillation.
    C. Asystole.
    D. Normal sinus rhythm.

108. When using a manual defibrillator, you should:

    A. Adjust the amplitude of the electrical signal to approximately four large squares on the graph paper.
    B. Place the electrode pads on the chest where you would normally place the defibrillation paddles.
    C. Suspect loose electrodes as the primary cause of artifacts.
    D. Use only the red and white patient monitoring cables for lead II observations.

109. Whether you are using a manual, automatic, or semi-automatic defibrillator, the initial countershock to an adult patient will be:

    A. 100 joules.
    B. 200 joules.
    C. 300 joules.
    D. 360 joules.

110. During the initial assessment phase of defibrillation, the first step is to:

    A. Discontinue CPR.
    B. Clear all personnel from contact with the patient.
    C. Attach the monitor leads to the patient.
    D. Discontinue chest compressions only.

111. In order to ensure that a countershock is actually delivered to the patient, the EMT should:

    A. Personally press the shock delivery switch.
    B. Observe the patient for sudden movement.
    C. Recheck the ECG after the shock for a deflection mark.
    D. Check the carotid pulse.

112. Called to the scene of a "man down, unknown cause," you find a female patient pulseless and apneic with no apparent signs of trauma. After performing quick-look, you identify the dysrhythmia as ventricular fibrillation. Following defibrillation, you note the patient's ECG display on the next page.

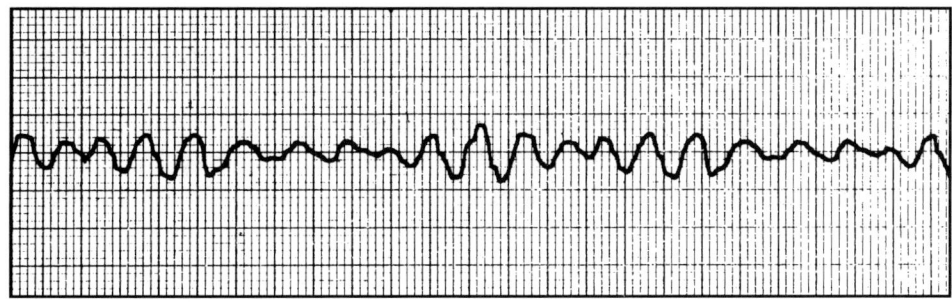

You would immediately:

   A. Repeat the defibrillation.
   B. Ascertain if a carotid pulse is present.
   C. Attach the ECG leads for further evaluation.
   D. Resume chest compressions.

113. Upon arriving at the scene of a medical emergency, you find a male patient in full arrest. Your partners begin CPR while you connect the defibrillator's patient monitoring leads. Analysis shows asystole and the patient is still pulseless. Next you should:

   A. Defibrillate at 200 joules.
   B. Defibrillate at 360 joules.
   C. Resume CPR.
   D. Discontinue resuscitation efforts.

You and two partners have been dispatched to the home of a 43-year-old female. Dispatch advises you en route that the patient stated that she had experienced a sudden onset of chest pain. History given to dispatch includes a recent hysterectomy approximately 12 days earlier and the patient complains that she hasn't felt well since the surgery. Dispatch further informs you that the patient's pain is nonradiating and is aggravated by respiration. Upon arrival at the scene you find the patient unresponsive, nonbreathing, and pulseless.

114. Your crew's first action should be to:

   A. Ventilate the patient.
   B. Attach the monitor leads.

C. Start chest compressions.
D. Turn on the defibrillator power.

115. Your crew has completed all of the activities listed as options in the previous question. Next, you direct your partners to clear the patient and begin assessment of the heart rhythm. Excessive artifact is noted so you should:

    A. Press the adhesive patches on the skin.
    B. Continue CPR.
    C. Unsnap the black monitor lead.
    D. Re-gel the defibrillator paddles.

116. After correcting the artifact problem noted in the previous question, you observe the following rhythm. You should:

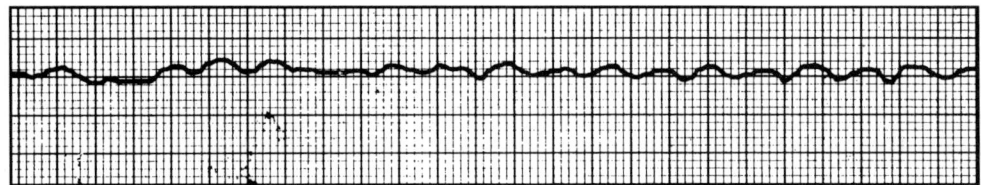

    A. Deliver up to three shocks.
    B. Resume CPR.
    C. Recheck the pulse.
    D. Cease resuscitative efforts.

117. Failure to deliver a defibrillatory shock when ventricular fibrillation exists is most often caused by:

    A. Insufficient charging time for the capacitors.
    B. Pressing the defibrillation buttons simultaneously.
    C. Excessive 60-cycle interference.
    D. Inadequately charged batteries.

Answers with Rationale

1. (A) The air we breathe usually contains about 20% oxygen, 79% nitrogen, and 1% minute amounts of other gases.

2. (C) Waste products are exchanged for oxygen and nutrients in the capillaries. The exchange of gases in the lungs takes place in the small capillaries located in the alveoli (air sacs).

3. (C) The epiglottis is the leaf-shaped valve that protects the trachea from food and liquids. The esophagus is found posterior to the trachea and is the passageway for food to the stomach. The larynx (voicebox) is the first part of the trachea. The pharynx is the throat.

4. (A) The cartilaginous rings of the trachea provide the shape and rigidity needed to keep the airway from collapsing during respiration. Crushing injuries to these rings can cause airway collapse and a life-threatening airway problem. A slight positive pressure is developed during exhalation.

5. (A) The muscles of the diaphragm and ribs both contract during inspiration, causing the diaphragm to flatten and the ribs to expand and rise, increasing the volume of the chest cavity and creating a slight negative pressure.

6. (B) Normally, carbon dioxide is the major blood gas stimuli for respiration. In some diseases, such as emphysema, this stimuli is replaced by the level of oxygen present in the arterial blood.

7. (D) The capillaries are located between the arterioles and venules. Blood flows from the arteries into arterioles, capillaries, venules, and then into veins.

8. (A) The visceral pleura covers the lungs. The parietal pleura lines the chest wall. The pleural space is just a very thin film of fluid between the visceral and parietal pleurae.

9. (A) The mediastinum is the space between the lungs. Should a shift be caused by lung injury, deviation of the trachea can be observed. Each half of the thorax is referred to as a hemithorax.

10. (D) The trachea, esophagus, thymus, connective tissue, and the heart and its large vessels are contained in the mediastinum.

11. (D) The nasopharynx is considered part of the upper airway and is posterior to the mouth and nose and superior-anterior to the esophagus and trachea.

12. (B) Metabolism is the chemical process by which life-maintaining energy is extracted from food. Catabolism is the destructive phase of metabolism. Epidemiology is the study of the relationships between host, agent, and environment in disease. Etiology is the study of the cause of the disease.

13. (A) The sticky, fluid part of the blood is plasma. A leukocyte (leukos = white and cyte = cell) is a white blood cell and combats infection. Platelets assist in blood clotting. Erythrocytes (erythro = red and cyte = cell) are the oxygen-carrying red blood cells.

14. (C) The septum divides the heart into two halves, each containing an atrium and ventricle. The mediastinum is a portion of the thoracic cavity between the pleural sacs containing the heart and its great vessels.

15. (C) The pulmonary artery and the aorta would be allowed to fill if the valves between the atria and ventricles were closed and the valves from the ventricles were open.

16. (B) Blood pumped out of the right side of the heart will enter the pulmonary artery. The pulmonary vein returns oxygenated blood from the lungs to the left atrium. The left ventricle fills the aorta. The great veins returning blood from the body to the right atrium are called venae cavae.

17. (D) The autonomic nervous system controls the diameter of the blood vessels. Arterial blood pressure is influenced by the size of the container (diameter of the blood vessels), the volume (blood) in the container, and the pump (heart) strength.

18. (B) We exhale approximately 16% oxygen, thus using only 4% to 5% oxygen out of the 20% available in the atmosphere.

19. (B) Tidal volume is the volume of air exchanged during respiration. The residual volume is what is left in the lungs after total exhalation. The vital capacity is a total of tidal volume and inspiratory and respiratory capacity.

20. (D) Brain death usually begins within four to six minutes after the brain is deprived of oxygen. If cardiac function remains for a period after ventilatory arrest, oxygen will be used in the lungs and will extend the period before brain death occurs. Other factors, including hypothermia and age, may slow or mitigate brain damage caused by cerebral hypoxia.

21. (A) Orthopnea is difficulty in breathing except when sitting or standing. Apnea is the absence of breathing. Dyspnea is labored breathing. Hypoxia is a lack of adequate oxygen content.

22. (D) Cardiac arrest would immediately deprive the brain of further oxygenation. With airway obstruction or pulmonary arrest, some oxygen remains in the lungs and is used before brain death occurs. Angina pectoris is chest pain caused by ischemia or lack of oxygen to the cardiac muscle.

23. (B) CPR may be discontinued if a physician assumes responsibility. Discontinuing CPR is a medical decision and should not be ceased even though police may instruct you to do so. Once you begin, you may cease CPR only if you become exhausted and cannot continue, or if you are relieved by another BLS provider.

24. (A) Verbal stimuli and a patient's response or lack thereof is the best indicator of unconsciousness. An unconscious patient's pupils may continue to react to light; opening the airway is not an appropriate stimulus. Pinching the lobe of the ear offers little in the way of pain stimuli.

25. (A) Rolling the unconscious patient can be made easier by bringing the patient's arm that is nearest you above his or her head and then gently rolling the patient, protecting the head and spine, until he or she is in a recovery position. This procedure can be done by one EMT.

26. (D) A partially occluded airway would still allow for respiratory effort. Retraction of intercostal and supraclavicular spaces would indicate respiratory effort. Snoring sounds could indicate the tongue resting against the throat.

27. (A) Forceful mouth-to-mouth ventilation should be used only as a last resort in clearing an airway obstruction. This action may blow an obstruction past the narrow point of the airway (larynx and epiglottis) and provide a partial airway.

28. (D) The jaw thrust maneuver is the best choice for opening an airway in a patient with a suspected neck injury. This can be done with the patient's neck and head in a neutral position, thus not further endangering the spine.

29. (A) Flexion of the neck will block the airway with the tongue. Try talking with your chin on your chest and observe the difficulty you experience. People with large necks may be difficult to hyperextend but may still have the airway adequately opened by use of the chin lift or jaw thrust.

30. (A) An adult should be artificially ventilated 10 to 12 times per minute; a child should be ventilated even more often.

31. (B) You should take four to ten seconds to check unresponsiveness in a patient who appears to be unconscious. Give him or her a chance to awaken and respond.

32. (D) After the airway is opened, allow three to five seconds for the patient to ventilate on his or her own. After five seconds, ventilate two times if respiration is not present.

33. (D) You should observe the rise and fall of the chest during each ventilation. Give two breaths of $1\,^1/_2$–2 seconds each. Slow inspiratory flow rate will avoid trapping air in the lungs between breaths and possibly prevent gastric distention, regurgitation, and aspiration.

34. (B) A patient with a stoma requires ventilation directly into the stoma or a tube if present. This is the laryngectomy's airway. Oral suction may not be required, as the upper airway is blocked either surgically or by a

trachea tube isolating it. Seal the patient's mouth and nose if you hear air escaping during mouth-to-stoma ventilation.

35. (B) A suction device should be ready when relieving severe gastric distention. Turn the patient onto his or her side and press between the xiphoid and umbilicus. A high degree of danger of aspiration exists, but severe distention must be relieved. Slower inspiratory flow rates or cricoid pressure may minimize the risk of gastric distention. Adequate ventilation usually does not need to exceed 1200 mL (1.2 L).

36. (D) The hands are placed between the xiphoid and slightly above the umbilicus in the Heimlich maneuver to relieve airway obstruction.

37. (C) Marked cardiac slowing may occur if the vagus nerve is stimulated. This can occur if the carotid body is overly stimulated while the carotid pulse is checked. Blood clots lodged in the neck may also be dislodged.

38. (D) The airway of an unconscious patient should be maintained by head tilt as the pulse is checked. It isn't necessary to pinch the nostrils unless you are ventilating. The hand behind the neck may not adequately maintain the open airway.

39. (D) The patient has a partial obstruction, probably caused by the tongue. Reposition the head and neck. He or she probably won't require artificial ventilation if the airway is corrected.

40. (C) The tongue is the most common type of airway obstruction. The tongue resting on the nasopharynx will cause a snoring sound. A complete airway obstruction will allow no air to pass and no sounds will be heard.

41. (C) Irreversible brain damage separates clinical from biological death. Biological death occurs four to six minutes after clinical death.

42. (A) Slow ventilations (1–1½ seconds each) sufficient to make the chest rise and fall should be delivered to an infant in respiratory arrest. The infant's neck should be kept in a neutral position even though overextension of the head has not been proven to collapse the trachea. Use a rate faster than for an adult while sealing both the infant's mouth and nose.

43. (B) Five to ten seconds should be used to establish pulselessness after ventilating a nonbreathing adult two times. This interval will allow time for proper location of the carotid pulse and for planning what to do next.

44. (B) The head tilt–chin lift maneuver creates the greatest opening for air passage. The safest first approach to opening the airway of a victim with a suspected neck injury is the jaw thrust technique, without head tilt.

45. (D) Reposition the head, as the tongue is the most likely airway obstruction. Again, attempt to ventilate.

46. (A) After repositioning the head and chin, apply subdiaphragmatic abdominal thrusts (up to five times) and again attempt to ventilate. Each new thrust should be a separate and distinct movement.

47. (C) After repositioning the head and chin, and applying up to five abdominal thrusts, using a hooking action, perform a finger sweep and then attempt to ventilate.

48. (B) The proper depth of compression for an adult is 1½" to 2" (3.8–5.0 cm).

49. (C) During chest compressions, 50% should be the downstroke and 50% the upstroke. Compression should be performed smoothly, without jabs. Chest compressions are performed with your arms pushing straight down while you rock at the hips

50. (D) Two-person CPR, performed on an adult, is performed at a ratio of five compressions to one ventilation. Pause between each set of compressions for a ventilation of 1½–2 seconds.

51. (C) Compressions performed on an adult by two rescuers should be delivered at a rate of between 80–100 per minute.

52. (D) When a second rescuer joins you in providing CPR, you should complete your series of 15 compressions.

53. (A) After you have completed your series of 15 compressions, check the victim for a spontaneous pulse.

54. (C) Bob Guy should now be positioned at the chest ready for you to give the patient one breath before he begins compressions.

55. (C) Bob Guy should begin compression at a rate of 80–100 per minute. You should provide one ventilation after each 5th compression. The ventilation should take 1½–2 seconds.

56. (A) During one-person CPR on an adult, you should deliver 15 compressions (9–11 seconds) and then two breaths (1½–2 seconds each), all in a period of 13–18 seconds.

57. (C) CPR may be interrupted for up to 30 seconds in order to move a patient downstairs or out of a hazardous location. Generally, 5 seconds is the limit. Keep in mind that each time CPR is stopped, blood pressure falls to zero.

58. (B) Children most often suffer pulmonary arrest (caused by airway obstruction) before cardiac arrest. Advanced stages of airway infection, such as croup, can occlude the airway and lead to death.

59. (B) When using the chin lift method of opening the airway of a child, you should keep the mouth open and not apply excess pressure on the soft tissues under the jaw, as this may close off the child's airway. If the child is unconscious, open the airway even if he or she shows no sign of cyanosis.

60. (D) Infants in need of artificial ventilation should be ventilated every three seconds, or 20 times per minute. Adults should be ventilated every five seconds, or 12 times per minute.

61. (A) Transport him immediately. Very likely this young patient has a progressive airway problem. Attempts to relieve a foreign-body obstruction will be useless and potentially dangerous.

62. (B) Foreign-body airway obstruction in an infant is handled by delivering a series of either five back blows and five chest thrusts or vice versa. Abdominal thrusts are not used because of the potential damage to underlying organs. Hyperextension of the neck is not needed to open the airway of an infant. Blind finger sweeps may push an object further down in the child, so they are not used.

63. (D) The brachial artery is the artery of choice in checking an infant under age 1 for pulselessness. The carotid is hard to find in the small, fat neck of an infant. Precordial motion may be an impulse rather than actually indicating cardiac output. The carotid artery is used in children over age 1.

64. (D) Infant CPR is performed by exerting pressure on the midsternum one finger width below a line drawn between the nipples. The heart of the infant is lower in the chest cavity than was previously thought.

65. (B) Compression depths between 1/2" and 1" (1.3–2.5 cm) are indicated for an infant.

66. (D) The compression rate for an infant is at least 100 times per minute. With pauses for ventilation, the ultimate number of compressions will actually be at least 80 per minute.

67. (B) CPR on infants and children is done at a five-to-one ratio. Children approximately age 8 and older are treated like an adult.

68. (C) Should you need to telephone for assistance, you should generally do this as soon as you determine the adult patient is unconscious. Infant and pediatric patients should receive one minute of CPR prior to telephoning for assistance.

69. (B) Properly performed chest compressions will produce peak pressure of 60–80 mmHg, but the mean pressure seldom exceeds 40 mmHg.

70. (A) The count "One, two, three . . ." is used for infant CPR to achieve 100 compressions per minute. "One and two and three . . ." will give you a rate of about 80 per minute for one- and two-rescuer child and adult CPR.

71. (A) Reassess your hand position, but do not stop CPR. Your fingers should not be on the chest wall at any time. Depth of compression must be maintained in order to squeeze the chest sufficiently to cause adequate blood flow.

72. (A) The carotid pulse should always be checked after the first minute of CPR. Artificial pulses should be palpable during chest compressions. It is used as an indicator of good profusion since it leads to the brain.

The femoral artery may also be checked for artificial and spontaneous pulses.

73. **(B)** The volume of air given during artificial ventilation should be just enough to cause the chest to rise. Any excess pressure will lead to gastric distention and possible lung damage. Each inspiratory rescue breath for an adult should be 1½–2 seconds. Adequate volume for an adult is 0.8–1.2 liters.

74. **(D)** A child or infant should be turned completely on his or her side to relieve gastric distention. Distention should be relieved only if it interferes with proper ventilation. Abdominal thrusts are dangerous when used on young children.

75. **(D)** A 50% concentration of oxygen can be obtained with the use of a pocket mask device with 10 liters per minute O_2. Up to an 80% concentration can be achieved with 15 L/min.

76. **(B)** You should maintain an airtight seal on the mouth and nose when using a pocket mask. A head tilt, chin or jaw lift is used to open the airway, and you should remove your mouth after each ventilation to get another breath.

77. **(C)** Oropharyngeal airways are used only on unconscious patients because gagging, retching, or vomiting may occur if the patient is awake.

78. **(D)** A lubricated oral airway should be inserted with a rotating motion to prevent pushing the tongue further back down the airway. If a tongue blade is used to move the tongue, the airway may be inserted without rotation. The patient's neck should be hyperextended unless contraindicated by suspected injury.

79. **(A)** The proper length for a nasopharyngeal airway can be estimated by selecting an airway that is the same length as the distance between the nose and earlobe. Always lubricate the airway prior to inserting it through the nostril. Follow the floor of the nose until the flange rests against the nostril.

80. **(B)** All bag-valve-mask systems should use transparent face masks in order to visualize the airway. Standard 15/22 mm fittings are used for

EOA and endotracheal tube connection. Sponge rubber in the bag is difficult to disinfect and may fragment.

81. (D) Water is necessary to clear the suction tip and tubing, as secretions are often sticky. Suction equipment should deliver 300 mmHg vacuum through large-bore tubing. Metal suction tips can damage the patient's teeth.

82. (D) Suction should be applied only after the tip is in place. (Close off "Y" tubing.) Continual suction removes available oxygen that the patient needs. Suction should be applied where needed. Disposable rubber gloves should be worn when suctioning patients.

83. (A) Frothy sputum generally indicates a lung condition such as contusion, pulmonary edema, or laceration of the airway.

84. (B) Tachycardia (fast heart rate) will be present in early hypoxia as the heart tries to compensate for the low oxygen tension. The patient will be nervous and irritable. Cyanosis is a later sign indicating poor perfusion.

85. (D) A chronic obstructive lung disease (COLD) patient may stop breathing as large concentrations of O_2 are introduced. Oxygen is a drug and should be treated as such. Oxygen will not burn or explode on its own. Oxygen toxicity occurs after many days of O_2 delivery.

86. (D) Medical gases are usually delivered to a patient at pressures between 40 and 70 psi. Steel gas cylinders are generally filled to between 2000 and 2200 psi.

87. (C) Never use a high-pressure cylinder without an O-ring or washer in place. Cracking the valve briefly before putting the regulator on will clear dust and debris from the opening. Never put oil or grease on oxygen fittings, because this may cause an explosion. Always face the gauge away from people when turning a tank on, as it may explode.

88. (C) The "safe residual" is always 200 psi. This prevents moisture and dirt from entering the cylinder.

89. (B) You should always see if a patient's nose is open before using nasal prongs. Simply occlude one nostril and then the other as the patient

breathes in with his or her mouth shut. You can expect concentrations of 35% to 50% O_2, and the flow rate will be set between 4 and 6 L/min.

90. (C) Simple face-mask O_2 delivery will use a flow rate between 6 and 10 L/min and deliver 35% to 60% O_2 concentrations. Humidified O_2 should be used any time delivery is expected to be prolonged (30–45 minutes). The face mask does not provide positive pressure and should not be used while performing CPR.

91. (B) The mask and bag can deliver 90% concentrations of O_2. Since the flow rate is adjusted so the bag is never fully collapsed or full, it can be used on adults or children.

92. (B) Venturi masks can deliver fairly accurate percentages of O_2. Masks are less comfortable for conscious patients, so cannulas are frequently used. Oxygen level will not be affected by the patient's rate or depth of respirations.

93. (D) The bag-valve-mask is of little use when performing CPR alone. Too much time is needed to maintain the oral airway, achieve a tight seal, and ventilate with only one EMT. An infant-sized bag holds 150–240 cc, best matched for the infant's small lung capacity. Reservoirs on the bag provide up to 100% O_2 concentrations. Resuscitation bags should not contain a pressure-relief valve. If one is present, the valve should be able to be manually bypassed to permit ventilation of a patient with poorly compliant lungs. The rate of ventilation for an infant should be between 40 and 60 per minute when using a bag-valve-mask device.

94. (A) The suction catheter should be passed only the distance between the mouth and earlobe. It is important to avoid gagging, which may stimulate vomiting. Remember: Never force the catheter, and apply suction only while the catheter is being removed.

95. (A) The proper way to measure an oral airway is to choose one that will reach from the lobe of the ear to the corner of the mouth. Longer airways can cause laryngeal spasms and/or vomiting. The airway is removed if the patient shows signs of gag reflex action.

96. (B) When nasal prongs are used, the patient is free to talk and relax without the anxiety associated with a face mask. Even mouth breathers

will benefit (as long as the nasal passages are open). Long O_2 delivery times should have humidification.

97. (D) A crushed larynx or trachea will best be cared for by encouraging the patient to take slow breaths, keeping the neck neutral, and administering O_2. Positive-pressure ventilation may actually increase the air in the surrounding tissue and compound the problem of subcutaneous emphysema.

98. (D) An oral airway that is too short may be of as little value as no airway at all and cause occlusion. Laryngeal spasms, vomiting, and gag reflex action often occur from the use of an oral airway that is too long.

99. (B) Oxygen humidifiers should be sterilized and the water should be changed after each use. Otherwise, a high degree of infection is possible to other patients. Humidifiers are probably the most neglected pieces of equipment on ambulances. For this reason, disposable humidification reservoirs are very desirable.

100. (B) The head should always be at the level of the heart or lower during CPR. Blood cannot reach the brain if the head is elevated above the level of the heart. The side rails of a cot are to protect the patient and are not meant for lifting.

101. (A) CPR should begin within 4–6 minutes after a patient's collapse if a cardiopulmonary resuscitation is to be successful. CPR should continue at all times for a cardiac arrest patient except during the assessment and treatment (defibrillation) cycles. Early defibrillation of collapse of a patient in ventricular fibrillation greatly improves patient outcome.

102. (D) In the normal heart, electrical impulses travel through a well-defined conduction pathway consisting of the SA node, AV junction, bundle of His, and the right and left bundle branches. The SA node, or sinoatrial node, is a cluster of specialized cells near the top of the right atrium and is the normal pacemaker of the heart.

103. (B) The QRS is the complex formed as the electrical impulse travels from the Purkinje fibers to the ventricles, causing both ventricles to contract. The T-wave is the deflection formed during the ventricular resting period. The P-wave is formed as the electrical impulses spread through the atria and cause both atriums to contract. The PR interval is

the time between the beginning of the P-wave to the beginning of the QRS complex.

104. **(D)** The ECG tracing shows a normal sinus rhythm. The heart rate is about 70 per minute. Each small (1 mm) block on the ECG paper represents 0.04 seconds. The larger boxes edged with bold lines represent five small boxes, or 0.20 seconds. Count the number of QRS complexes in 6 seconds and multiply the number by 10 to establish the rate. The heart rhythm shown is regular since the distance between each QRS complex is the same. The rhythm is supraventricular since the QRS complex is 0.12 seconds or less.

105. **(C)** When assessing a patient believed to be in ventricular fibrillation (VF), it is always important to check the patient for pulselessness. It is imperative to always treat the patient, not the ECG rhythm. A patient in VF will be pulseless. A patient in ventricular tachycardia may have a palpable pulse but will generally deteriorate to VF within 60 seconds of onset. Asystole (standstill) is the final rhythm of the heart and follows ventricular fibrillation.

106. **(A)** The ECG shows ventricular tachycardia (VT). The beats originating in the ventricles are broad, slurred, and slightly distorted. The rate shown is approximately 170 beats per minute and there is little variation in height or rate. Automatic defibrillators generally will not countershock ventricular tachycardia, which can rapidly deteriorate into VF.

107. **(B)** The ECG shows ventricular fibrillation. The overall pattern of the strip is irregularly shaped, chaotic, and lacks any regular repeating features. The height of the electrical signal and distance between the peaks of the signal vary greatly in VF.

108. **(C)** An artifact is caused by outside interference with the ECG and sometimes resembles VF. Loose electrodes caused by contact with oily, dirty, or diaphoretic skin can result in artifacts. Chest hair and dried gel on the pads can also cause poor signal transmission. An unsnapped cable will produce a straight-line tracing. The amplitude of the ECG should be adjusted to approximately two large blocks on the ECG paper. Placement of electrodes on the chest must be done in such a manner as to not interfere with defibrillation paddle placement.

109. **(B)** The initial countershock, whether delivered by an automatic or manual defibrillator, will be given at 200 joules or watt-seconds. Subsequent countershocks should be delivered according to orders previously set by your Medical Director.

110. **(C)** During the initial assessment phase of defibrillation, monitor leads or defibrillator pads must be connected to the patient. Once the leads are in place and the device is turned on, discontinue CPR and clear all personnel from contact with the patient. Cable movement, agonal respirations, or muscle tremors can interrupt rhythm interpretation and CPR should be resumed until the rhythm can be adequately assessed.

111. **(B)** All EMTs must recognize the sudden movement of the patient that indicates the countershock has been delivered. Prior to either type of defibrillation device shocking the patient, all personnel must be clear of the patient, including any contact the EMTs might have with the ambulance cot or metal spineboards. Automatic and semi-automatic defibrillators generally require about 15 seconds to analyze and charge prior to either countershock or giving the operator a "shock advised" signal. Repeat "shock" each time the message screen on a semi-automatic device displays "shock advised" until a total of three shocks in a row have been delivered. If a pulse does not return, resume CPR.

112. **(B)** Prior to defibrillating VF a second time, you must make certain that the patient does not have a pulse. Poor paddle-to-skin contact during a quick-look may produce artifact that mimics VF. That is one reason why many protocols allow for ECG interpretation of rhythms only through patient monitoring cables. Once it has been verified that the patient remained pulseless, the paddles are recharged and defibrillation is repeated at 200–300 joules depending on local protocol. A third countershock would be delivered at 360 joules.

113. **(C)** If the rhythm is asystole and no pulse is present, direct your partners to resume CPR and check to be sure that the problem is not with your equipment. Keep in mind a disconnected patient cable lead can present a straight-line tracing. Check the connections at the patient and at the monitor. If using a manual defibrillator, you should ensure that the lead selector is in the lead II position. Then check for possible hidden VF by assessing the rhythm for five seconds in lead I and then five seconds in lead III. Countershock if VF is observed in any lead.

114. (A) Your team's first action for care of this patient is to begin CPR. Two ventilations are given followed by chest compressions. Ventilations should be delivered through the use of a bag-valve-mask device using 100% oxygen. The third member of the crew could then turn the defibrillator power on, turn the recorder on, begin the verbal report, and attach the monitor leads or defibrillator pads. The history given should cause you to suspect pulmonary embolism as the underlying malady.

115. (A) Excessive artifact can be caused by several conditions including unsnapped or loose patient cables. Press monitor patches against the patient's skin to ensure firm contact. CPR must be discontinued only during the rhythm assessment. Rhythm should be interpreted through the use of patient monitoring cables and not the quick-look feature of defibrillator paddles.

116. (C) The patient's pulse must be checked after each activity you perform. If she is still pulseless and her ECG shows ventricular fibrillation, countershock would be in order. Generally, your Medical Control will have established a protocol to deliver up to three shocks to a patient in VF. Energy levels used for defibrillation will also be prescribed by your Medical Control.

117. (D) Most often inadequately charged batteries or batteries that have spontaneously discharged will prevent the delivery of a shock when VF exists. Defibrillator batteries, including backup units, should be checked for adequate charge daily and after each use. Insufficient capacitor charging time can also cause failure to deliver a shock, but occurs less often than battery problems.

6 Wounds, Bleeding and Shock

Chapter 6 stresses the recognition and treatment of open and closed soft-tissue injuries, bleeding and its control and, most important, shock. Certifying agencies traditionally devote 10% to 20% of their written exams to these topics.

All body organs require a continuous supply of blood to furnish oxygen and nutrients. Disruption of this flow is potentially dangerous, and the EMT is frequently called upon to deal with a bleeding injury. Included here are such topics as gunshot wounds, crush injuries, and amputations as well as bandaging and control of bleeding.

Although use of the pneumatic counter-pressure device is currently under debate, this topic is included for review by EMTs working in EMS systems using PCPDs. This device is also known as a Pneumatic Anti-Shock Garment (PASG) and as a Medical Anti-Shock Trouser (MAST).

EMTs are reminded to use appropriate precautions to reduce the potential for exposure to bloodborne diseases. Body Substance Isolation techniques are intended to prevent parenteral, mucous membrane, and nonintact skin exposure of health care workers to bloodborne pathogens. The type of protective attire should be appropriate to the procedures to be performed. Vinyl or latex gloves should be available for health care workers who wish to use them. Always follow current CDC guidelines and applicable state or local regulations regarding the handling and disposal of infectious waste.

1. What is the average number of liters of blood usually found in the adult cardiovascular system?

   A. Three.
   B. Four.
   C. Six.
   D. Seven.

2. Shock can be caused by all of the following conditions except:

   A. Heart damage.
   B. Blood vessel constriction.
   C. Loss of blood volume.
   D. Blood vessel dilation.

3. Which of the following conditions is usually present when a person is in shock?

   A. High urinary output.
   B. Slow pulse.
   C. Slow respirations.
   D. Cool skin.

4. Which of the organs listed below can survive longest without adequate perfusion?

   A. Skeletal muscle.
   B. Kidney.
   C. Spinal cord.
   D. Gastrointestinal tract.

5. The term *perfusion* means the circulation of blood through or within the:

   A. Veins.
   B. Arteries.
   C. Capillaries.
   D. Organs.

6. Hemorrhagic shock is also termed:

   A. Cardiogenic shock.
   B. Neurogenic shock.

C. Septic shock.
D. Hypovolemic shock.

7. Mr. Durfee has been involved in a head-on automobile accident. He has been thrown through the windshield, and you find him lying on the ground. His appearance leads you to believe he is in shock. Which type of shock can you most likely rule out?

   A. Hemorrhagic.
   B. Respiratory.
   C. Neurogenic.
   D. Psychogenic.

8. Your initial care for Mr. Durfee would be to check his:

   A. Pulse.
   B. Blood pressure.
   C. Cervical spine.
   D. Airway.

9. Transfusion of blood, elevation of the legs, and use of a pneumatic counter-pressure device is not particularly helpful in what kind of shock?

   A. Cardiogenic.
   B. Hemorrhagic.
   C. Hypovolemic.
   D. Neurogenic.

10. Full inflation of the pneumatic counter-pressure device is indicated in the treatment of:

    A. Pelvic fractures.
    B. Pulmonary edema.
    C. Vaginal bleeding in pregnancy.
    D. Isolated head injuries.

11. Mrs. Alevaras has been ill for several days with uncontrollable diarrhea and vomiting. Her blood pressure is 70/40 and she appears to be very anxious. You should expect to find the following:

    A. Strong pulse.
    B. Rapid pulse.

C. Slow respirations.
D. Moist skin.

12. You should suspect Mrs. Alevaras is in shock, the type of which is:

    A. Septic.
    B. Metabolic.
    C. Neurogenic.
    D. Cardiogenic.

13. Your general care for Mrs. Alevaras should include:

    A. Elevating her lower extremities.
    B. Administering fluids orally for rehydration.
    C. Recording vitals at 20-minute intervals.
    D. Promoting the loss of body heat.

14. Additional care for Mrs. Alevaras should include:

    A. Administration of low-concentration O_2.
    B. Use of heating pads using the ambulance AC converter.
    C. Reassurance.
    D. Administration of her hypertension medications.

15. Which of the following injuries leads to shock first?

    A. Fractured tibia.
    B. Fractured humerus.
    C. Three-inch laceration of the upper arm.
    D. Ruptured spleen.

16. Mr. Ward has been involved in an industrial accident at a petroleum refinery. Several 55-gallon drums have pinned him in a sitting position. A drum is crushing his right chest. His left lower arm appears to be fractured. There is little external bleeding, but he appears to be in shock. Which type of shock is most likely the problem?

    A. Neurogenic.
    B. Respiratory.
    C. Cardiogenic.
    D. Hemorrhagic.

17. The drums cannot be moved off Mr. Ward until a forklift is readied. Your initial care for him should be to:

    A. Elevate his legs.
    B. Start O$_2$.
    C. Cover his abrasions with dressings.
    D. Splint his fractured arm.

18. Which type of shock could cause a temporary period of vascular dilation?

    A. Psychogenic.
    B. Neurogenic.
    C. Cardiogenic.
    D. Hemorrhagic.

19. General signs of shock can include:

    A. Diaphoresis.
    B. Cherry-red skin color.
    C. Slow, shallow respirations.
    D. Lustrous eyes and constricted pupils.

20. Additional signs of shock include:

    A. Nausea and vomiting.
    B. Restfulness.
    C. Hot, dry skin.
    D. Lack of thirst.

21. A common sign or symptom present during anaphylactic shock is a:

    A. Stable blood pressure.
    B. Cherry-red skin color.
    C. Bounding pulse.
    D. Wheezing sound during exhalation.

22. Anaphylactic shock can be caused by:

    A. Rapid deceleration in a motor vehicle accident.
    B. Gunshots.
    C. Inhaled substances.
    D. Exposure to X-ray.

23. Select a possible symptom of anaphylactic shock:

    A. Hypertension.
    B. Slow pulse rate.
    C. Cherry-red skin color.
    D. Laryngeal edema.

24. Treatment for anaphylaxis includes:

    A. High-concentration O_2.
    B. Elevation of the upper torso.
    C. Encouraging the patient to keep physically active.
    D. Injection of 1:10,000 epinephrine.

25. You are called to an MVA and find a patient lying unconscious next to a car. Your patient has an apparent closed fracture of the tibia and an open fracture of a humerus with moderate bleeding. After establishing an open airway and the presence of a pulse (120), your first action should be to:

    A. Administer O_2.
    B. Stop the obvious bleeding.
    C. Splint the fractured tibia.
    D. Elevate the legs.

26. After the care rendered in Question 25, you should:

    A. Administer O_2.
    B. Stop the obvious bleeding.
    C. Splint the fractured tibia.
    D. Elevate the legs.

27. Having completed the care in Questions 25 and 26, you should then:

    A. Administer O_2.
    B. Stop the obvious bleeding.
    C. Splint the fractured tibia.
    D. Elevate the legs.

28. When treating a patient believed to be in hemorrhagic shock, you should:

    A. Elevate the thighs with the knees bent.
    B. Elevate the patient's head.

C. Place patient in supine position with legs elevated no more than 12 inches.
D. Not use positive-pressure ventilation if the legs are elevated.

29. In caring for a patient who has experienced psychogenic shock, your primary activity should be to:

    A. Elevate the feet.
    B. Start O_2.
    C. Examine for injuries caused by falling.
    D. Prevent loss of body heat.

30. The most effective means of controlling external bleeding of an extremity is the use of:

    A. Direct pressure.
    B. Pressure points.
    C. Tourniquets.
    D. Elevation.

31. A person can donate a pint of blood without significant problems. A person losing a pint of blood from trauma may go into shock. What one factor may be responsible for the difference in reactions?

    A. Rate of blood loss.
    B. Posture of patient in whom blood is lost.
    C. Arterial blood loss.
    D. Venous blood loss.

32. Normal clotting time for blood is about:

    A. 1–2 minutes.
    B. 2–5 minutes.
    C. 6–10 minutes.
    D. 10–15 minutes.

33. External bleeding from a capillary will:

    A. Spurt and be bright red.
    B. Spurt and be dark bluish-red.
    C. Ooze and be bright red.
    D. Ooze and be dark bluish-red.

34. Mr. Garcia has a large laceration on his left thigh. It is bleeding bluish-red blood and is flowing out at a moderate rate. You should suspect Mr. Garcia to be bleeding mainly from:

    A. Arteries.
    B. Veins.
    C. Capillaries.
    D. Arterioles.

35. Your first action in controlling Mr. Garcia's bleeding should be to:

    A. Apply direct pressure to the wound.
    B. Apply pressure at the femoral artery.
    C. Apply a tourniquet.
    D. Take his vital signs.

36. After applying a sterile dressing to Mr. Garcia's thigh, you see by the blood-soaked dressing that the bleeding has not yet been controlled. You should now:

    A. Remove the dressing and observe.
    B. Apply pressure to the femoral artery.
    C. Apply a tourniquet.
    D. Apply more pressure by hand.

37. When used alone, the pressure-point method of controlling bleeding is often unsuccessful because of the:

    A. Difficulty in locating the proper point.
    B. Presence of collateral circulation.
    C. Need to remove patient's clothing.
    D. Additional discomfort experienced by the patient.

38. Tourniquets are used only as a last resort to control bleeding because they:

    A. Are difficult to apply.
    B. Must be released every 20 minutes.
    C. Can be used only below the elbow or knee.
    D. Cause considerable nerve and tissue damage.

Wounds, Bleeding, and Shock

39. Excessive blood loss, either external or internal, may produce shock in all patients. Choose the danger level of blood loss.

    A. Adult loss of more than 300 mL of blood.
    B. Adult loss of more than 500 mL of blood.
    C. School-age child loss of more than 300 mL of blood.
    D. Infant loss of more than 30 mL of blood.

40. Applying a splint to external bleeding best aids the control of bleeding by:

    A. Immobilizing the long bone.
    B. Aiding in venous return.
    C. Preventing contamination of the wound.
    D. Aiding clotting through immobilization of the tissue.

41. The term used for vomiting of bright red blood is:

    A. Epistaxis.
    B. Hematuria.
    C. Hematochezia.
    D. Hematemesis.

42. During an altercation, Robert Wilder was hit in the face with a fist. When you arrive, you find that he is bleeding heavily from his nose and spitting blood. His blood pressure is 110/70. Your care for Mr. Wilder should include:

    A. Laying the patient on his back.
    B. Pinching his nostrils.
    C. Applying warm packs to his nose.
    D. No attempt to control his bleeding.

43. During the course of treatment and transportation of Mr. Wilder, you should expect:

    A. A sharp rise in blood pressure.
    B. Hematemesis.
    C. Increased bleeding if O_2 is administered.
    D. Little change in the amount of bleeding.

44. Internal bleeding may be suspected if a patient experiences a rapid pulse and:

    A. Melena.
    B. Slow respirations.
    C. Stable blood pressure readings.
    D. Warm, dry skin.

45. Mr. Schwartz has a pulse of 140 and blood pressure of 90/60. He is complaining of sharp pains in his stomach. There is no evidence of trauma. You should care for Mr. Schwartz by:

    A. Giving ice water to relieve pain.
    B. Administering O_2.
    C. Transporting Mr. Schwartz in a prone position.
    D. Applying ice to his belly.

46. The skin has many bodily functions. Choose the correct statement.

    A. Temperature changes in the environment are recognized by the epidermis.
    B. The dermis is the first layer of defense against the admission of bacteria.
    C. The dermis is the watertight layer of skin.
    D. The nerves that convey environmental temperature changes are located in the dermis.

47. A black-and-blue mark on the skin is also called:

    A. Ecchymosis.
    B. Urticaria.
    C. Hematoma.
    D. Petechiae.

48. A lump caused by a pool of blood from a fracture or contusion is a/an:

    A. Ecchymosis.
    B. Urticaria.
    C. Hematoma.
    D. Hemolysis.

49. Blood in the urine is called:

    A. Epistaxis.
    B. Hematuria.
    C. Hematochezia.
    D. Hematemesis.

50. Initial management for closed soft-tissue injuries of an extremity include the:

    A. Use of proximal pressure points.
    B. Application of ice packs.
    C. Lowering of the extremity below the heart.
    D. Use of a board splint for immobilization.

51. A soft-tissue injury that is normally caused by scraping and presents oozing blood would be classified as a/an:

    A. Abrasion.
    B. Laceration.
    C. Avulsion.
    D. Puncture.

52. Amputated tissue can best be cared for by:

    A. Immersion in saline solution.
    B. Freezing.
    C. Wrapping in sterile gauze and cooling.
    D. Wrapping in sterile gauze and warming.

53. The first action in the treatment of open soft-tissue wounds should be to:

    A. Prevent further contamination.
    B. Control bleeding.
    C. Immobilize the injured area.
    D. Remove any embedded material.

54. Care for a patient with a piercing foreign object should include:

    A. Applying direct pressure on the object to control bleeding.
    B. Using minimal dressings in order to allow constant observation.
    C. Cutting the object off as close to the skin as possible.
    D. Leaving the object in place and immobilizing it.

55. When using a pressure dressing and bandage on an extremity, it is always important to:

   A. Use sterile materials.
   B. Splint even the small lesions.
   C. Use soft roller bandages.
   D. Check distal circulation after bandaging.

56. An open wound with jagged or smooth edges is classified as a/an:

   A. Abrasion.
   B. Avulsion.
   C. Laceration.
   D. Puncture.

57. From the following list of organs, which is/are the first to experience reduced blood flow due to shock?

   A. Skin.
   B. Muscles.
   C. Heart.
   D. Intestines.

58. The best indicator of blood circulation for a patient in shock is the:

   A. Level of consciousness.
   B. Pulse rate.
   C. Urinary output.
   D. Respiratory rate.

59. A patient whose motor response withdraws from painful stimuli would receive a Glascow Coma score of:

   A. 6.
   B. 5.
   C. 4.
   D. 3.

60. What is the Champion/Sacco trauma score for a systolic blood pressure of 50–69 mmHg?

   A. 4.
   B. 3.

C. 2.
D. 1.

61. A Glascow Coma score between 11 and 13 would be converted to a Champion/Sacco trauma score of:

    A. 5.
    B. 4.
    C. 3.
    D. 2.

62. During the examination of a patient suspected of having internal bleeding, you obtain a pulse and blood pressure with the patient lying down. You then sit the patient up to recheck the vitals and find the pulse rate has increased 20 beats per minute and the blood pressure has fallen 20 mmHg. You can conclude that the patient:

    A. Is frightened.
    B. Has lost at least 1 unit of blood.
    C. Is orthopneic.
    D. Is in cardiogenic shock.

63. While examining an adult patient in shock, you can palpate the femoral pulse but not the radial pulse. You estimate the minimum systolic blood pressure to be:

    A. 50 mmHg.
    B. 70 mmHg.
    C. 90 mmHg.
    D. 110 mmHg.

64. Choose the signs which best represent a patient who has reached an advanced level of shock:

    A. Pale skin, rapid and weak pulse.
    B. Cyanotic skin, rapid and weak pulse.
    C. Pale skin, slow and weak pulse.
    D. Cyanotic skin, rapid and strong pulse.

65. A patient with abdominal organs protruding from a laceration to the body would best be cared for by:

    A. Replacing the organs in the abdomen.

B. Covering the organs with a dry, sterile dressing.
C. Wrapping the patient in a burn sheet.
D. Covering the organs with a sterile dressing and moistening it with saline solution.

66. Bill Hollis has caught his arm in a piece of heavy machinery, which crushes and nearly tears it off. Bleeding is minimal considering the extent of injury. The arm is attached only by some soft tissue and skin and will surely be surgically amputated. Your care should include:

    A. Completing the amputation in order to apply pressure on the stump.
    B. Packing the forearm in ice.
    C. Using a tourniquet on the stump.
    D. Straightening the skin flap or bridge, avoiding pressure dressings on the bridge.

67. After removing a crushed ring from a finger, you should:

    A. Elevate the finger and apply heat.
    B. Elevate the finger and apply cold packs.
    C. Lower the finger and apply soap.
    D. Lower the finger and apply cold packs.

68. A high-pressure injection injury can occur from mishandling compressed air tools. Which statement best describes the result of a high-pressure injection injury?

    A. Bleeding is usually bright red.
    B. Bleeding is usually very heavy.
    C. Little swelling is noted but person appears in shock.
    D. Rapid swelling occurs from edema.

69. Called to a home, you find a small child with his hand stuck in a toy. Care for the child's clamping injury should include:

    A. Applying pressure on the brachial artery.
    B. Applying green soap to the hand and elevating it above the head while removing the toy.
    C. Applying petroleum jelly to the hand and stepping on the toy while removing it.
    D. Transporting the child to the Emergency Department for extrication.

70. Choose the correct statement regarding gunshot wounds.

    A. The size of the bullet is more important than its velocity.
    B. The bullet that passes all the way through a patient will cause less damage than one that does not.
    C. The shape of a bullet has little influence on tissue damage.
    D. Entrance wounds are typically bigger than exit wounds.

71. Gunshot wounds to the head may require special treatment including:

    A. Tight pressure dressings to control bleeding.
    B. Ice packs over facial wounds.
    C. Removal of foreign objects or debris impaled in the wound.
    D. More direct pressure on exit wounds.

72. Proper care for a gunshot wound to the neck includes:

    A. Tight pressure dressings around the neck.
    B. Elevation of the head to reduce bleeding at the neck.
    C. Avoidance of the use of suction equipment.
    D. Immobilization of the head and spine.

73. Perhaps the most important part of your care for a patient who has suffered stab wounds is to:

    A. Cover all wounds with sterile dressings.
    B. Use only local pressure to control bleeding.
    C. Immobilize the injured extremity.
    D. Recognize potential damage to underlying organs.

74. Randy Conyer has been involved in a MVA. He is demonstrating the classic signs and symptoms of shock. His systolic and diastolic pressures have dropped. He responds only to painful stimuli. Considering the signs and symptoms, what percentage of blood volume would you suspect the patient has lost?

    A. 40% or more.
    B. 30–35%.
    C. 20–25%.
    D. Less than 15%.

75. What percentage of a patient's available blood volume can be translocated with the proper application of a pneumatic counter-pressure device?

    A. 5%.
    B. 10%.
    C. 30%.
    D. 50%.

76. You should inflate a pneumatic counter-pressure device until the:

    A. Pressure causes each compartment to be firm when squeezed.
    B. Pressure in the abdominal compartment is greater than the pressure in each leg compartment.
    C. Velcro starts to crackle.
    D. Patient's systolic BP is approximately 100 mmHg.

77. A pneumatic counter-pressure device can be used for:

    A. Controlling bleeding in the chest.
    B. Splinting of fractures involving only the legs.
    C. Controlling internal bleeding from a fractured pelvis.
    D. Reducing pulmonary edema.

78. A patient should have a PCPD inflated when he or she presents a clinical picture of shock and a systolic blood pressure at or below:

    A. 60 mmHg.
    B. 70 mmHg.
    C. 90 mmHg.
    D. 110 mmHg.

79. Relative contraindications to the use of a PCPD include:

    A. Intracranial bleeding.
    B. Intrathoracic bleeding.
    C. Long transport times.
    D. Cardiogenic shock.

80. The proper inflation procedure for a PCPD is to inflate:

    A. Both legs simultaneously and then the abdominal compartment.
    B. One leg at a time to maximum and then the abdominal compartment.

C. The abdominal compartment and then one leg at a time.
D. The abdominal compartment to 60 mmHg and then both leg compartments to 70 mmHg.

81. Proper positioning of a pneumatic counter-pressure device calls for the:

    A. Top of the abdominal compartment to be at the patient's umbilicus.
    B. Top of the abdominal compartment to be at the bottom of the lowest rib.
    C. Crotch of the pants to be pulled snugly around the patient's crotch.
    D. Bottom of the leg compartments to be even with the ankles.

82. The proper valve position of each compartment is essential to proper inflation and maintenance of device pressure. Select the correct valve positions with regard to activity.

    A. All valves are open during inflation.
    B. The abdominal compartment valve is closed when the leg compartments are being adjusted.
    C. All valves remain open once the device is inflated.
    D. Both leg compartment valves are always kept in the same position.

83. Although pneumatic counter-pressure devices are not deflated in the field, the EMT should know the proper steps of deflation in case the hospital staff is unfamiliar with the device. Choose the correct statement below regarding deflation.

    A. Deflation can be done in about 5 minutes while 100% O_2 is being administered.
    B. The abdominal compartment can be deflated for examination several times without risk to the patient.
    C. The abdominal compartment can be deflated and opened in the O.R. if the surgeon is prepared for rapid bleeding.
    D. All of the compartments must be deflated simultaneously.

84. Should the pressure gauge indicate a loss of pressure in a pneumatic counter-pressure device, you should:

    A. Check each compartment individually to determine which one is leaking.

B. Keep pumping the foot pump with all compartment valves open.
C. Discontinue the use of the garment, as all compartments must function properly.
D. Reduce the pressure in each compartment until each is equal with the leaking compartment.

85. After inflation of a PCPD, the desired patient blood pressure should be about:

   A. 70–80 mmHg.
   B. 90–110 mmHg.
   C. 110–120 mmHg.
   D. 120–130 mmHg.

86. Inflation of the PCPD on an average adult male in shock could produce improvements similar to the infusion of how much blood?

   A. 1 unit (500 mL).
   B. 2 units (1000 mL).
   C. 2½ units (1250 mL).
   D. 4 units (2000 mL).

87. Once the patient's blood pressure has reached the acceptable level, you should:

   A. Increase the PCPD pressure by 10 mmHg.
   B. Lower the PCPD pressure by 10 mmHg.
   C. Lower the PCPD pressure by 20 mmHg.
   D. Maintain the PCPD pressure or increase it if the patient's blood pressure begins to fall.

88. Select the sign or symptom that differentiates cardiogenic shock from hypovolemic shock.

   A. Chest pain.
   B. Rapid, regular pulse.
   C. Cool, moist skin.
   D. Reduced level of consciousness.

89. A patient with pulmonary edema will have:

    A. Flat neck veins.
    B. Crackling lung sounds (rales).
    C. A desire to lie flat while breathing.
    D. Slow, deep respirations.

90. Select the most correct statement regarding the application of a PCPD:

    A. A PCPD can be used on an obese patient.
    B. A PCPD cannot be used on a pregnant patient.
    C. A PCPD can be used on a patient with wet lungs.
    D. A PCPD can be used on a patient with an isolated head injury.

Answers with Rationale

1. (C) The average adult cardiovascular system contains 5 to 6 liters of blood so answer C is the closest. The loss of even 1 liter can have a profound effect on the patient.

2. (B) Constriction of blood vessels reduces the size of the cardiovascular container and thus increases available volume. This action would be desirable for a patient in shock and is often accomplished through the use of medications.

3. (D) The skin of a patient in shock will usually be pale, ashen, cool, and moist. Urinary output is reduced due to poor perfusion. The pulse rises in rate and becomes weak in quality (thready). Respiration rate increases as the respiratory system tries to adjust for the hypoxia present. A fall in the blood pressure is a later sign of shock.

4. (D) The gastrointestinal tract can survive longest without adequate perfusion. When in shock, the body will shunt blood away from digestive processes to support vital organs.

5. (D) Perfusion is the circulation of blood through organs. In perfusion, the blood travels through arteries, capillaries, and veins.

6. (D) Hemorrhagic shock is often referred to as hypo (lessened or lowered) volemic (volume) shock. Loss of blood in hemorrhagic shock reduces blood volume. Septic shock is caused by bacteria attacking the small blood vessel walls so that they loose plasma and blood and can no longer constrict. Neurogenic shock is caused by a loss of control by the nervous system to constrict the blood vessels. If the blood vessels dilate, there will be insufficient blood to fill the circulatory system.

7. (D) Psychogenic shock can be ruled out in Mr. Durfee's case, as he is lying on the ground and would have adequate blood supply returned if he had suffered syncope (fainting). The trauma received from the accident could lead to any of the other shock conditions listed.

8. (D) The first rule in treating any patient is to check and maintain the airway. Care must also be taken to protect the trauma patient's spine while opening the airway. Administer oxygen as indicated.

9. (A) Cardiogenic shock is a condition resulting from the inability of the heart to pump a patient's blood. This patient may be most comfortable if transported in a sitting position. Oxygen would be of benefit.

10. (A) Pelvic fractures can be immobilized and bleeding reduced through the use of pneumatic counter-pressure devices. Pulmonary edema is aggravated by the use of these devices. Head injury alone presents a rise in blood pressure—a sudden drop indicates other bleeding or near-death in a head injury patient. Inflation of the leg compartments of a PCPD may be beneficial for a pregnant patient experiencing vaginal bleeding if signs of shock are present.

11. (B) Mrs. Alevaras will probably have a rapid pulse rate. The pulse will be weak, the skin will be dry due to her dehydrated state, and respiration rate and depth will be increased.

12. (B) Metabolic shock, more commonly termed hypovolemic shock due to reduced fluid volume, should be suspected in Mrs. Alevaras' case. Her loss of fluid through diarrhea and vomiting has dehydrated her and resulted in decreased blood volume due to fluid loss.

13. (A) You should elevate the legs of Mrs. Alevaras to increase venous return. Fluid should not be given orally to a person in shock. Vitals should be recorded at 5-minute intervals. Body heat should be maintained at present temperature.

14. (C) Mrs. Alevaras should be reassured that she is in good hands while en route to the hospital. High-concentration O_2 is indicated. The use of heating pads is contraindicated since her reduced blood supply to the skin may predispose her to burns if heat is added. Oral administration of medications is also contraindicated.

15. (D) A rupture of the spleen causes a tremendous internal blood loss that can rapidly produce signs of shock. Tenderness over the upper left quadrant and pain in the left shoulder may be a clue to bleeding from the spleen.

16. **(B)** Mr. Ward is probably in respiratory shock, as he is unable to adequately oxygenate himself because of the drum crushing his chest. He may also be in hemorrhagic shock from associated internal bleeding.

17. **(B)** Initial care for Mr. Ward should be to start O_2, as his level of oxygenation to the blood has been reduced. Elevation of the legs would do little to reduce shock through venous return, as he is sitting up. After starting O_2, control bleeding and immobilize his fractures.

18. **(A)** Psychogenic shock is nothing more than a common faint or syncope. It is only a temporary condition that is relieved when the patient is placed in supine position and blood flow to the brain is re-established.

19. **(A)** Diaphoresis (profuse sweating) is common in shock. The skin color will first be pale or ashen, later becoming cyanotic. Respirations will normally be deep and rapid. The eyes will be lusterless and dull.

20. **(A)** As nerve control over the blood vessels is lost, the blood vessels in the abdomen dilate, causing nausea and vomiting. The patient will also be restless and thirsty and have cool, clammy skin.

21. **(D)** Wheezing sounds during exhalation are common during anaphylactic shock. This is caused by the constriction of the smaller bronchi. The skin may be flushing, itching, or covered with hives. The pulse will be weak and the blood pressure may fall drastically.

22. **(C)** Anaphylactic shock is a severe allergic reaction and can be caused by drugs, insect stings, foods, and inhaled substances.

23. **(D)** Anaphylaxis is initially characterized by flushing of the skin; itching of the eyes, mouth, or ears; rapid pulse; hypotension; bronchospasm; or laryngeal edema. It can progress rapidly to shock with cyanosis and unconsciousness.

24. **(A)** Treatment for anaphylaxis includes high-concentration O_2 and keeping the patient as quiet as possible. Avoid extraneous movements if the cause is an injected substance. Epinephrine (1:1000) may be injected subcutaneously if you are authorized by state or local protocol and directed to do so by your Medical Control. Treat hypotension with elevation of legs, etc.

25. (A) You should administer O₂ to all patients who are in shock or could go into shock. This should be done as early in the course of treatment as possible.

26. (B) After starting O₂, you should then stop any obvious bleeding. This action should include pressure dressing and splinting of the patient's open humerus fracture.

27. (C) After your care of the fractured humerus and airway, you should next splint the fractured tibia and then elevate the legs to encourage venous return.

28. (C) Hemorrhagic shock can be cared for by placing the patient in a supine position with legs elevated. The legs should not be elevated over 12 inches, nor should the knees be bent, trapping the blood distal to them. A patient may experience some additional difficulty breathing if the foot of a backboard is elevated since the abdominal organs will shift toward the thorax. Positive-pressure ventilation may be needed to assist this patient's breathing.

29. (C) A person who has fainted requires little or no care unless injured by a fall. Head injuries are quite common occurrences in fainting episodes and the patient should be examined for head injuries if recovery isn't rapid and complete. The patient may also need food or sugar.

30. (A) Direct pressure is the most effective way of controlling bleeding. It can be augmented by elevating the wound above the level of the heart. Pressure points only slow bleeding, as collateral circulation is almost always present. Tourniquets are seldom needed.

31. (A) The rate of blood loss is the factor that prevents a person donating blood from going into shock. During blood donation, the body's normal protective responses have time to constrict vessels and redistribute needed blood to the vital organs without compromise to them.

32. (C) Normal clotting time is 6 to 10 minutes. Direct pressure may be required to control bleeding until the blood clots.

33. (C) Capillary bleeding will ooze and be bright red, as the blood has yet to give off its oxygen. Spurting bright red blood is from arteries.

34. (B) Mr. Garcia's bleeding is primarily from veins. The bluish-red color is deoxygenated blood. The flow indicates venous pressure rather than spurts from an artery.

35. (A) Direct pressure on Mr. Garcia's wound should be your first action. The bleeding should be controlled without much difficulty, as it is venous bleeding.

36. (D) Should bleeding still be present, apply more dressings and pressure to the thigh. The dressings act as a matrix for coagulation. The pressure controls the flow. Do not remove dressings, as you will dislodge clots already formed and increase bleeding. Pressure points or tourniquets are not indicated.

37. (B) The presence of collateral circulation reduces the effectiveness of arterial pressure points by allowing blood to flow through secondary vessels when the primary is blocked. Direct pressure and elevation should be used in addition to pressure points to control stubborn bleeding.

38. (D) Tourniquets are used only as a last resort because they oftentimes crush a considerable amount of tissue beneath them, causing permanent damage. Once applied, they should not be removed until the patient is in the care of a physician. Tourniquets should not be used below the elbow or knee because of the additional potential of damage to these tissues, as nerves are closer to the surface of the skin. Seldom is bleeding so profuse that direct pressure and elevation cannot control it in these regions.

39. (D) Blood loss of 25 or 30 mL may cause an infant to go into shock. A child can tolerate blood losses nearing 500 mL, while an adult can lose up to 1 liter before shock becomes a threat.

40. (D) A splint may be used to control external bleeding by immobilizing the injured tissue. An air splint, blood pressure cuff, pneumatic counter-pressure device (PCPD), or vacuum splint may aid this process by placing direct pressure on and around the wound, promoting clotting and reducing blood supply.

41. (D) Hematemesis (hema = blood/emesis = vomiting) is vomiting of bright red blood. Epistaxis is bleeding from the nose. Hematuria is blood in the urine; hematochezia is blood from the rectum.

42. (B) Pinch Mr. Wilder's nose to control bleeding, or place a bandage between his gum and upper lip and press it. He should not lie down, as this will encourage aspiration of the blood in his throat. Ice packs may be helpful in controlling bleeding by causing vasoconstriction.

43. (B) It would not be unusual for Mr. Wilder to vomit blood (hematemesis) during your course of care. Much blood is swallowed when a person has a bloody nose. Vital signs may begin to point toward shock if bleeding persists, in which case O_2 should be administered to reduce the chance of hypoxia.

44. (A) Melena is the passage of dark or black stools which may indicate blood that has come in contact with the acids found in the digestive tract. Respirations will increase, and blood pressure may fall from internal bleeding, as it may lead to shock.

45. (B) Mr. Schwartz is showing signs of shock possibly caused by internal bleeding in the abdomen. Administration of O_2 is always indicated in shock. Transportation will probably be best in a shock position. Ice on the belly will do little to control the bleeding. Nothing should be given orally.

46. (D) The nerves of the skin are located in the dermis and convey environmental temperature changes to the brain. The epidermis is the watertight layer of skin that prevents the admission of bacteria.

47. (A) Ecchymosis is caused by extravasation of blood into the skin and is generally blue-black in color, later changing to greenish-brown or yellow. Urticaria are hives. Petechiae are small, purplish hemorrhagic spots on the skin.

48. (C) A hematoma (hema = blood/oma = tumor) is a lump created by a pool of blood caused by either crushing soft-tissue injury or fractures.

49. (B) Hematuria (hema = blood/uria = urine) is a term used to describe blood in the urine.

50. (B) Application of ice packs to closed soft-tissue injuries may help to control swelling of tissue. Splinting with an air splint will produce even pressure and may aid in the control of bleeding. A board splint may not be as useful, as the pressure exerted will not be even. Elevation of an extremity may also aid in reducing swelling and bleeding.

51. (A) An abrasion is usually caused by scraping of skin, as in a slide on pavement. An abrasion will ooze blood unless it is very deep. An avulsion can be either a partial or complete tear of tissue leaving a "flap" or an amputation.

52. (C) Amputated tissue should be wrapped in saline-moistened, sterile gauze, placed in a plastic bag, and then put on ice. Be sure not to freeze the part—only keep it cool. Do not immerse the part in any solution or apply a tourniquet to it.

53. (B) Your first action in the treatment of open soft-tissue wounds should be to control bleeding. Prevention of further contamination and immobilization should follow the control of bleeding. Do not spend time trying to remove embedded material.

54. (D) A piercing object should be left in place and immobilized unless it is penetrating the skin less than one millimeter. Large, bulky dressings can help to stabilize the object. Direct pressure around the object (but not against sharp edges) will help to control bleeding. If the object is exceptionally long, it may be cut off several inches above the skin. Remember that this action will cause vibration and increase bleeding.

55. (D) After applying a pressure dressing and bandage, you should always check the distal circulation to ensure that the bandage is not too tight. Numbness and tingling will present within just a few minutes if circulation is occluded. Sterile dressings are preferred, but use any clean material available to control bleeding. Soft roller bandages are very convenient to work with, but triangular bandages are a good standby.

56. (C) An open wound with either smooth or jagged edges is classified as a laceration. Puncture wounds are generally made with pointed objects or gunshots. The depth of this type of wound is hard to determine and may be much more serious than the bleeding might lead you to believe.

57. **(A)** The skin is the first organ of the body to experience reduced blood supply during shock. The body's autonomic nervous system shunts the blood away from the skin by causing peripheral vasoconstriction. In later stages of shock, this autonomic system fails because of hypoxia, and the vessels dilate, aggravating the volume-depleted situation even more.

58. **(A)** The level of consciousness of a patient in shock is an excellent indicator of whether or not the brain is being adequately perfused. Urinary output is difficult to check in the field as the patient should be catheterized. The pulse rate may remain stable for a period of time.

59. **(C)** A patient's motor responses are scored in the following manner. Obeys command, 6; localizes pain, 5; withdraws (pain), 4; flexion (pain), 3; extension (pain), 2; none, 1.

60. **(C)** Systolic blood pressure receives the following Champion/Sacco trauma score points: 90 mmHg or above, 4; 70–89 mmHg, 3; 50–69 mmHg, 2; 0–49 mmHg, 1; no pulse, 0.

61. **(B)** The total Glascow Coma score is converted to a Champion/Sacco trauma score by being divided by approximately one-third. A Glascow score of 11 to 13 would receive a trauma score of 4.

62. **(B)** Postural blood pressure and pulse readings that change, lowering 20 mmHg or rising 20 beats per minute, are significant. This is an excellent indicator that the patient has lost at least 1 unit of blood.

63. **(B)** A femoral pulse can usually be palpated if the systolic BP is 70 mmHg or more. Radial pulses may diminish if the systolic pressure is less than 80 or 90 mmHg.

64. **(B)** A patient in shock who starts to exhibit cyanosis of the skin, nailbeds, or lips has probably reached an advanced state of shock. The pulse will be weak and rapid, perhaps not even perceptible. The vessels themselves are no longer adequately perfused and thus dilate and exhibit cyanosis. That is not to say he or she cannot be saved through vigorous resuscitative efforts. Patients in an irreversible state of shock are usually yellowish-white due to a total lack of perfusion to the skin.

65. (D) Protruding abdominal organs should not be replaced while in the field. They should be covered with sterile dressings moistened with saline solution, and then covered with aluminum foil. This procedure keeps the organs moist and warm because the foil reflects and preserves body heat.

66. (D) Bill Hollis' mangled arm should be straightened at the skin bridge and the partial stump covered with a pressure dressing. Do not complete the amputation, as some tissue may be saved and used to cover the stump in surgery.

67. (B) After removing a crushed ring from a finger, elevate the finger and apply cold packs to reduce swelling. Seldom is heat used in the first 48 hours following an injury.

68. (D) Rapid swelling is common, but bleeding is usually minimal. A high-pressure injection wound is generally in a class by itself even though it may resemble a puncture wound.

69. (B) Clamping injuries, such as a child's hand stuck in a toy, can be relieved by applying a lubricant such as green soap or petroleum jelly and elevating the body part prior to attempting to remove the toy. The longer the patient is clamped, the more likely it is that swelling will increase and make extrication more difficult. Be careful not to do further injury such as degloving the patient. Ice or cold water may also help reduce swelling.

70. (B) Bullets that do not pass all the way through the patient often cause more damage than ones that do because the body absorbs the entire energy. Small-caliber bullets often tumble and bounce around, doing tremendous internal damage but causing little external bleeding. Bullets of different shapes (hollow points, wad cutter, etc.) can cause tremendous soft-tissue damage. Exit wounds are typically bigger than entrance wounds.

71. (B) Ice packs may be helpful in reducing edema in facial gunshot wounds. Loose bandages should be used on head injuries to provide a matrix for clotting. Do not use pressure dressings to stop bleeding in these cases because intracranial pressures may be increased, causing more damage.

72. (D) A patient with a gunshot wound of the neck should be placed on a spineboard and treated as though a spinal injury exists. Be sure to observe for any signs of paralysis or respiratory distress. Bleeding should be controlled with direct pressure, but do not wrap the neck. Elevation of the head would reduce blood supply to the brain and increase the potential of embolisms. Aggressive suctioning will be required in most of these patients.

73. (D) Stab wounds are often of unknown depth, and although the puncture or laceration through the skin may be dramatic, damage to underlying nerves, vessels, and organs may be of far greater concern. All wounds should be covered and bleeding should be controlled with pressure dressings. Seldom will a tourniquet be needed. Always remove all the clothing and examine carefully for hidden wounds, as there may be a life-threatening wound left undetected (e.g., sucking chest wound).

74. (B) Mr. Conyer's probable blood loss is in the 30–35% range. Coma occurs after about a 40% blood loss. A patient in a coma will not react to painful stimuli. A blood loss of 15% or less may not present any clinical signs of shock. A loss of 20–25% is demonstrated by increased pulse rate and a rise in the diastolic pressure as the body attempts to compensate.

75. (A) Studies have shown that no more than 5% of a patient's available blood supply is translocated by proper application of a pneumatic counter-pressure device. Significant improvements in blood pressure after inflation of the PCPD are believed to be caused primarily by increased peripheral vascular resistance rather than earlier beliefs about 30% blood volume translocation.

76. (D) The patient's blood pressure indicates the amount of inflation required of the pneumatic counter-pressure device. The pressure should be elevated in two stages to approximately 100 mmHg. The first level of inflation should be around 60 mmHg in each compartment, or until the Velcro begins to crackle. This occurs at about 60 mmHg. Then you should recheck the BP. If the pressure has not risen to accepted levels, continue inflation to 100 mmHg, or until the pop-off valves release.

77. (C) A PCPD can effectively control internal bleeding from pelvic and proximal femur fractures. Pelvic and hip fractures may also be immobi-

lized through the use of the PCPD. The PCPD will probably aggravate pulmonary edema.

78. (C) A patient presenting the clinical signs of shock (rapid pulse and respirations; cool, clammy skin; anxiety; etc.) and a systolic BP of 90 mmHg or less should have a PCPD applied unless contraindications exist.

79. (D) Cardiogenic shock is a relative contraindication to the use of the PCPD. When signs of shock are present, use is indicated even in head or chest injury, and when relatively long transport times are anticipated.

80. (A) The proper inflation sequence is to inflate both leg compartments simultaneously to 60 mmHg (or when Velcro crackles) and close the leg valves. Then inflate the abdominal compartment to 60 mmHg and check the patient's BP. If it has risen to approximately 100 mmHg, do not inflate further. If the BP has not reached the acceptable level, continue to inflate legs first and then the abdominal compartment to 100 mmHg or until pop-off valves release (104 mmHg).

81. (B) The proper positioning of a PCPD calls for the top border of the abdominal compartment to be just below the 12th ribline. Placement above this level will seriously compromise the patient's ability to breathe.

82. (B) During inflation of the PCPD, the leg compartments are opened together and the abdominal compartment is shut. After the legs are inflated to 60 mmHg, the valves are closed before the abdominal valve is opened. All valves are closed after the device is inflated. If a drop of pressure is suspected, each compartment can be checked separately and reinflated.

83. (C) The abdominal compartment can be deflated in the operating room if the surgeon is prepared to control bleeding immediately. The legs can remain inflated and the abdominal compartment reinflated after surgery. The patient usually requires infusion of large quantities of IV solutions before deflation can begin. The process commonly takes 30–45 minutes, slowly releasing pressure 5–10 mmHg at a time, and restabilizing the patient with fluids before another release of pressure.

84. (A) Should the pressure gauge indicate a loss, check each compartment individually for a leak. Reinflate to previous pressure. The device can still be of value even if a section fails.

85. (B) The acceptable blood pressure level of a patient being cared for through the use of a PCPD is a systolic pressure between 100 and 110 mmHg. Do not overinflate, as this will actually increase the bleeding.

86. (B) When the PCPD is properly inflated, the average adult male will experience improvement in his clinical outlook similar to those experienced with the infusion of 2 units (1000 mL) of blood. This improvement is caused primarily by increased peripheral vascular resistance.

87. (D) Once the patient's blood pressure has reached the acceptable level (100–110 mmHg systolic), you should maintain the PCPD pressure as is or increase to maximum if the patient's BP falls below the accepted level.

88. (A) Cardiogenic shock will present with many of the common signs of hypovolemic shock, as well as possible chest pains from acute MI or pulmonary edema. This is a complex medical emergency for the BLS EMT to handle.

89. (B) A patient with pulmonary edema will have crackling lung sounds (rales). The neck veins may be distended; respirations will be rapid and shallow. The patient will desire to sit up to ease his or her breathing. Pulmonary edema is a contraindication for the use of a PCPD.

90. (A) A PCPD can be used on a obese patient even if the abdominal compartment cannot be closed and filled. The pressure exerted by the filled leg compartments will benefit the patient. The same is true of a patient in an advanced stage of pregnancy. Wet lungs (rales) indicates the presence of pulmonary edema, a contraindication to the use of a PCPD. A patient with an isolated head injury will probably have an elevated BP.

7 Musculoskeletal System

This chapter is designed to help the EMT review the basic anatomy (muscles and bones) of the body. The questions on immobilization not only review the procedures necessary to properly immobilize fractures but also point out some of the many complications that can arise from injury to or improper handling of the skeletal system. Attention will be given to inflatable, rigid, and traction splints and use of short and long spineboards. Some questions relate to the use of pneumatic counter-pressure devices as they apply to fractures.

Across the United States, certifying bodies dedicate 10% to 15% of their written exams to these topics. Application of these skills represents an even larger percentage of material tested in practical exams.

1. What is the name of the oily, clear fluid that nourishes and lubricates articular cartilage?

    A. Seminal fluid.
    B. Amniotic fluid.
    C. Epithelial fluid.
    D. Synovial fluid.

2. The orbit (eye socket) includes which one of the following bones:

    A. Zygoma.
    B. Temporal.
    C. Mandible.
    D. Parietal.

3. The acetabulum is found at the:

    A. Shoulder.
    B. Elbow.
    C. Knee.
    D. Hip.

4. The small wrist bones, just distal to the ulna and radius, are the:

    A. Metacarpals.
    B. Carpals.
    C. Phalanges.
    D. Metatarsals.

5. The lateral end of the clavicle is part of the:

    A. Glenoid fossa.
    B. Acromioclavicular joint.
    C. Sternoclavicular joint.
    D. Glenohumeral joint.

6. How many vertebrae are found in the cervical spine?

    A. 4.
    B. 5.
    C. 7.
    D. 12.

7. The tough, ropelike cords that attach muscles to bones are:

    A. Aponeuroses.
    B. Tendons.
    C. Ligaments.
    D. Striates.

8. The prominences at one or both ends of the bone, normally serving as attachment points for ligaments, are called the:

    A. Condyles.
    B. Trochanters.
    C. Epiphyseal plates.
    D. Heads.

9. Select the phrase that best describes a closed fracture.

    A. Bone deformity and a puncture wound just above the deformity.
    B. Bone deformity, with no evidence of a break in the skin.
    C. Bone deformity, with a large wound and bone fragments visible.
    D. Little deformity, with wound visible near the site of pain.

10. Open wounds associated with fractures should:

    A. Have area cleansed with Betadine and then splinted in the position found.
    B. Be covered with moist, sterile dressings.
    C. Have bleeding controlled by tourniquets.
    D. Be covered with dry, sterile dressings and aligned to facilitate splints.

11. Which of the following is the most reliable sign of an underlying fracture?

    A. Point tenderness.
    B. Swelling.
    C. Ecchymosis.
    D. A patient's guarding or refusing to move an extremity.

12. Sprains and dislocations are types of injuries involving joints. Select the sign or symptom that may be seen in a dislocation but not in a sprain.

    A. Deformity.

B. Tenderness.
C. Swelling.
D. Loss of some function.

13. During your examination of a patient suspected of having a fracture involving a limb, before splinting you should:

    A. Remove patient's clothing in cases of open fractures.
    B. Ask the patient to move the injured limb through its full range of motion.
    C. Evaluate presence and quality of the distal pulse and nerve function.
    D. Avoid palpating the limb if the patient complains of generalized pain throughout the limb.

14. When examining a patient suspected of having fractures of the lower extremities, you should check for loss of sensation in the:

    A. Anterolateral aspect of the thigh.
    B. Dorsolateral aspect of the foot.
    C. Proximal portion of the lower extremity.
    D. Little toe.

15. Initial care of a severely deformed limb should include:

    A. Straightening with manual traction.
    B. Splinting in place if distal pulse is absent.
    C. Splinting in place, immobilizing the joint above and below the fracture.
    D. Straightening all deformities regardless of patient discomfort, as it is only temporary.

16. The most important rule to be followed during the application of rigid splints is to:

    A. Apply the splints to only the lateral and medial aspects of the limb.
    B. Pad the splint to fill in any hollow spots.
    C. Use elastic bandages to attach the splint.
    D. Support the limb and apply traction until the splint is completely applied.

17. Which statement is most correct regarding air splints?

    A. Air splints can apply pressure on open wounds.
    B. Large air splints should be inflated with a foot pump.
    C. Air splints are unaffected by temperature or altitude changes.
    D. Air splints are ideal for fractures of the humerus.

18. Most traction splints can be applied:

    A. On arms or legs.
    B. Inside pneumatic counter-pressure devices (PCPD).
    C. Only if patient's foot gear remains on the patient.
    D. On leg fractures involving the femur, hip, or lower leg.

19. During the transportation of a patient with fractures, you should:

    A. Keep patients with upper-extremity fractures lying flat.
    B. Elevate the extremity when lower-extremity fractures are present.
    C. Apply hot packs to fractures.
    D. Rapidly transport all fracture patients, using red lights and siren.

20. Which of the following is not an essential step in evaluating a patient with injured extremities?

    A. General assessment of the patient.
    B. Visual examination of the limbs.
    C. Neurovascular evaluation distal to the injury.
    D. Range-of-motion examination of affected limbs.

21. Select the neurovascular exam results indicating a severe dysfunction below the level of a fracture.

    A. Capillary filling in two seconds.
    B. Distal pulse palpable below injury.
    C. Tingling on the dorsal side of the foot or hand.
    D. Inability to dorsiflex foot or hand.

22. A "blowout" fracture that often causes the eye to look down and limits eye motion in other directions involves the:

    A. Mandible.
    B. Maxilla.

C. Nasal bone.
D. Mastoid.

23. The clavicle is considered part of the:

    A. Thorax.
    B. Shoulder girdle.
    C. Neck.
    D. Arm.

24. Fractures involving the clavicle or scapula should be immobilized by the use of a:

    A. Figure-eight bandage.
    B. Backboard.
    C. Sling and swathe.
    D. Pillow splint.

25. Proper field care for a dislocated shoulder should include:

    A. Reduction of the dislocation.
    B. Transportation in a supine position.
    C. Splinting by use of pillows and sling.
    D. Application of hot packs to increase circulation.

26. Splinting of a fractured humerus:

    A. Can be achieved by using gentle traction and applying a sling and swathe.
    B. Should only be done using board splints.
    C. Should be applied in the position found if the distal pulse is absent.
    D. Should be accomplished using a traction splint.

27. Select the most appropriate statement regarding injuries to the elbow.

    A. Sprains of the elbow joint are more frequent than dislocation of the elbow.
    B. Swelling is seldom seen in a dislocated elbow.
    C. An epiphyseal fracture is of greater concern in adults than in children.
    D. The greatest danger of an elbow injury is that of nerve or blood vessel damage.

28. Proper care of a fractured elbow includes:

    A. Splinting in place if distal pulse is present.
    B. Splinting with the elbow at a 90° angle and hand slightly raised, regardless of distal circulation.
    C. No change of position if distal pulse is absent, as further movement may sever vessels.
    D. Aggressive straightening of the joint to re-establish distal pulse when absent in position found.

29. A fracture of the ulna or radius shaft should be cared for by immobilizing the:

    A. Wrist.
    B. Elbow.
    C. Wrist and elbow.
    D. Hand, wrist, elbow, and shoulder.

30. Select a type of splint that should not be used on a severely angulated fracture of the lower arm that has a good distal pulse:

    A. Full arm air splint.
    B. Ladder splint.
    C. SAM splint.
    D. Vacuum splint.

31. A "Colles fracture" involves the:

    A. Carpal bones.
    B. Radius.
    C. Humerus.
    D. Radius and ulna.

32. Proper care for injuries involving the hands includes:

    A. Applying bulky dressings with the hand in the position of function.
    B. Popping dislocated fingers back into place.
    C. Immobilizing suspected fractures and hanging the hand dependent to reduce pain and swelling.
    D. Packing the hand in ice to reduce swelling.

33. The best management for a patient with a severe pelvic fracture with severe hypotension is the application of:

    A. One traction splint.
    B. Pneumatic counter-pressure device.
    C. Long spineboard.
    D. Two traction splints.

34. Severe bleeding from a pelvic fracture is:

    A. Seldom seen.
    B. Seen only with open wounds.
    C. Usually into the pelvic cavity and retroperitoneal space.
    D. Usually into the thigh.

35. Select the most appropriate statement about hip dislocation injuries.

    A. The sciatic nerve is most often injured in anterior dislocations of the hip.
    B. An anterior hip dislocation will present with the knee drawn up and the thigh rotated in and adducted.
    C. An anterior hip dislocation is usually caused by a direct forward blow to the knees when a patient is sitting (as in a car).
    D. Traction splints should not be applied to dislocated hip injuries.

36. An elderly patient with an isolated fracture of the proximal femur can be:

    A. Diagnosed if the injured leg is shorter and turned in.
    B. Immobilized by placing the patient on a spineboard and placing pillows around the limb for support.
    C. Treated with a traction splint set at 50 pounds torque.
    D. Placed in a pneumatic counter-pressure device inflated to 140 mmHg.

37. When caring for a patient with a severe injury to the knee, you should:

    A. Splint in place if distal pulses are strong.
    B. Repeatedly attempt to straighten the knee if distal pulses are absent.

C. Apply a traction splint to reduce the dislocation if distal pulses are absent.
D. Apply gentle traction while straightening the knee even in cases where the patient feels increased pain.

38. After determining that your patient, Mr. Schubert, has suffered a mid-shaft fracture of the femur, you should:

   A. Splint in place if no distal pulse is observed.
   B. Gently apply traction, straighten the leg, and apply an air splint.
   C. Apply a traction splint and recheck distal pulse and nerve status.
   D. Apply a pneumatic counter-pressure device over a Hare traction splint.

39. The most frequently fractured bone in the body is the:

   A. Radius.
   B. Fibula.
   C. Scapula.
   D. Clavicle.

40. You are called to an apartment building fire. When you arrive, you are directed to a 24-year-old male patient who has jumped from a third-floor balcony. He is complaining of pain in both heels. You should:

   A. Pillow-splint both feet and transport the patient in a level, supine position.
   B. Air splint both feet and let the patient sit with his legs straight.
   C. Pillow-splint both feet and transport on a spineboard with the feet slightly elevated.
   D. Apply rigid splints to both feet and apply a cervical collar to the patient's neck.

41. From the choices below, select the most reliable symptom of spinal injury in a conscious patient.

   A. Painful movement.
   B. Lower extremities cool to the touch.
   C. Complaint of pain or numbness in the spine.
   D. Weakness on one side of the body.

42. During your examination of a female motor vehicle accident victim who is conscious, you attempt to determine the presence of a spinal injury. The last step of examination you would perform is to:

   A. Ask about pain, weakness, or tingling in the lower extremities.
   B. Have the patient move her fingers and toes.
   C. Have the patient move her spine to see if movement produces pain.
   D. Feel for a deformity or tenderness along the spine.

43. Local policy may or may not call for the removal of helmets from patients with suspected neck injuries. Select the most appropriate statement regarding helmet removal.

   A. The helmet need not be removed if the airway can be easily maintained.
   B. The chin strap should be cut while traction is applied to the helmet.
   C. The helmet should slide off the patient's head with little effort after the chin strap is cut.
   D. Full-face helmets must be tipped forward to facilitate removal.

44. Proper care for a suspected spinal injury patient should include:

   A. Splinting the neck in the position found if the airway is adequate.
   B. Always splinting the neck in an "eyes-forward" position if no resistance is felt.
   C. Release of manual traction once a cervical collar is applied.
   D. Application of a chin strap to immobilize the head to a spineboard.

45. The two most common complications of spinal cord injury are:

   A. Hypovolemic shock and cardiac arrest.
   B. Neurogenic shock and ventricular fibrillation.
   C. Hemorrhagic shock and failure of the hypothalamus.
   D. Neurogenic shock and paralysis of chest muscles.

46. A tingling or pricking sensation is termed:

   A. Paresthesia.
   B. Priapism.

C. Porphyria.
D. Peristalsis.

47. You have performed a primary survey on a trauma patient and have decided to load him into the ambulance and transport due to a BP of 80/40 and uncontrollable bleeding from a large leg wound. En route to the hospital, you perform a secondary examination on the unconscious patient. After examining his head and neck, you would then check his:

    A. Shoulders.
    B. Arms.
    C. Abdomen.
    D. Pelvis.

48. A properly immobilized fracture of the humerus should not allow movement at the:

    A. Wrist.
    B. Elbow and wrist.
    C. Shoulder and elbow.
    D. Shoulder and wrist.

49. Traction splints should be applied to:

    A. Crushing injuries of the lower limbs.
    B. Dislocated knees.
    C. Fractured femurs.
    D. Fractures of the ankles.

50. When immobilizing a patient on a short or long spineboard, you should:

    A. Immobilize the trunk before the head.
    B. Release manual neck traction after a foam cervical collar is applied.
    C. Apply chin straps if available.
    D. Straighten the patient's legs after all straps are firmly in place when transferring to a long board.

51. When applying most traction splints, you should:

    A. Adjust the splint length after it is placed under the patient.

B. Remove the patient's shoes and socks before splinting.
C. Apply traction before fastening the ischial strap.
D. Grasp the ankle only when applying manual traction without a commercial hitch.

52. Occasionally, an injury to muscle tissue may cause swelling that is limited by the intermuscular septum. As an emergent concern, one can rule out:

    A. Compromise of nerve function.
    B. Compromise of the muscles.
    C. Compromise of the circulation.
    D. Bone dysfunction.

53. Proper care for a spinal injury patient demonstrating signs of neurogenic shock includes:

    A. Elevating the head and shoulders to aid breathing.
    B. Elevating the foot of the spineboard 8 to 12 inches.
    C. Elevating the foot of the spineboard at least 16 inches.
    D. Lowering the foot of the spineboard about 6 inches.

54. Peroneal nerve damage will cause the patient to be unable to:

    A. Flex the knee joint.
    B. Dorsiflex the foot.
    C. Feel sensation on the medial surface of the foot.
    D. "Grip" with the toes.

55. Examination of the patellas reveals that they are both on the same level. You can generally rule out all of the following injuries except:

    A. Hip fractures.
    B. Femoral fractures.
    C. Dislocated hip.
    D. Tibial fracture.

56. The average blood loss for patients with fractures involving the pelvis is:

    A. 1000–3000 cc.
    B. 500–1000 cc.

C. 250–600 cc.
D. 50–250 cc.

57. Select the sign or symptom that would differentiate between pelvic fractures and hip fractures.

   A. Inability to move the leg.
   B. Pain felt upon pelvic compression.
   C. Pain in proximal leg or hip.
   D. Crepitus.

Answers with Rationale

1. (D) Synovial fluid is the clear, oily lubricant found in articulating joints. Seminal fluid is the male fertilizing fluid. Amniotic fluid surrounds the fetus in the uterus as a protective mechanism. The epithelial tissues are the cells that form the outer surface of the body.

2. (A) The orbit (eye socket) includes the zygoma and maxilla. The mandible is the lower jaw bone. The parietal and temporal bones are part of the skull.

3. (D) The acetabulum is the socket portion of the hip formed by the innominate bones.

4. (B) The carpal bones are the small wrist bones. The phalanges are the fingers. The metacarpals are the small bones of the hand found between the phalanges and carpals. The metatarsals are found in the foot.

5. (B) The lateral end of the clavicle is part of the acromioclavicular joint. The glenoid fossa is the recess for the articulation of the humeral head. It allows lateral movement. The sternoclavicular joint is composed of the medial end of the clavicle and the sternum. The glenohumeral joint is the true shoulder joint.

6. (C) There are 7 cervical vertebrae. There are 4 coccyx and 5 lumbar vertebrae. The thoracic vertebrae number 12.

7. (B) Tendons are tough, ropelike cords that attach muscles to bones. Aponeuroses are broad, fibrous sheets attaching muscles to one another. Ligaments attach bones to bones.

8. (A) Condyles are prominences found at one or both ends of long bones. Trochanters are projections where tendons insert into bones. Epiphyseal plates are transverse cartilage plates that allow for bone growth.

9. (B) A closed fracture is one in which there is no break in the skin. It may also be called a simple fracture. All fractures with open wounds (compound), whether or not the bone is visible, are considered to be open fractures.

10. (D) Compound (open) fractures should have the wounds dressed with dry, sterile dressings. These fractures can be realigned by applying gentle traction to facilitate splinting. Tourniquets are seldom needed to control bleeding from broken bones. If resistance or increased pain is noted, splint in the position found. Treatment protocols may vary by jurisdiction.

11. (A) Point tenderness is the most reliable sign of an underlying fracture. Swelling may be present in other injuries. Rapid swelling with a doughlike resilience is a sign of bleeding. Ecchymosis may take several hours to appear. A patient's guarding or refusing to move an extremity is a strong sign of some type of injury, not just a fracture.

12. (A) A sprain or dislocation can present with tenderness, swelling, and possible loss of function. A dislocation may have joint deformity, while a sprain will not.

13. (C) All patients suspected of having a fracture should have distal pulse and nerve status evaluated before and after splinting. Clothing, including shoes and socks, should be removed in cases of suspected fractures to facilitate adequate visual examination. Capillary refilling and ability to move the extremity in both planes are important signs. Palpation of a limb can localize a fracture site. Patients should not be encouraged to move limbs if pain exists.

14. (B) Nerve damage to the lower leg can often be determined by a sensory exam of the dorsolateral aspect of the foot and the great toe. The patient may complain of numbness or tingling. Even the slightest change in sensation is an important finding.

15. (A) Severely deformed extremities should be straightened to near normal alignment. This will often increase blood flow and reduce patient discomfort. If moving the limb causes extreme pain, splint it in place. Recheck distal neurovascular status after splinting. If pulse is lost, contact Medical Control, as they may direct you to loosen or reposition the splints.

16. (D) Always support the injured limb and apply gentle traction until the splinting process is completed. Secure the proximal end of the splint first. It does no good to immobilize the distal end of a broken bone first.

Splints should be padded, not only to fill voids but also to protect all body surfaces they contact. Soft roller bandages may be used to wrap splints. Avoid the use of elastic bandage wraps in the field, as their use may compromise circulation.

17. (A) Air splints can apply direct, even pressure to the limb to which they are applied. Air splints are never inflated with a foot pump. They are affected by changes in altitude (air ambulance) and temperature (from cold environment to warm ambulance). Air splints do not properly immobilize fractures above the level of the elbow or knee, as the proximal joint is not incorporated into the splint. Proper inflation is checked by depressing the splint with the thumb. It should depress somewhat but not so much that it can easily touch the inner surface (next to the patient).

18. (D) A traction splint may be used for leg fractures not involving the knee or ankle. Much less traction is required for a tibia/fibula fracture than that involving the femur. Traction splints should not be used on upper-extremity fractures, as undue force would be applied to the axilla. Foot gear should be removed to facilitate proper examination of the distal neurovascular status. Most traction splints cannot be applied inside a pneumatic counter-pressure device.

19. (B) Fractures involving the lower extremities should be raised slightly during transportation of the patient. This action will help reduce swelling and combat shock. Ice packs (not on bare skin) will also aid in the reduction of swelling and pain. Few fractures are life-or-death situations; thus, the use of red lights and siren is not indicated.

20. (D) Range-of-motion examinations are not essential in the evaluation of extremity fractures. General patient assessment, including airway and signs of shock, should precede the visual examination of the injured limbs. Distal pulse and nerve status must always be determined before and after splinting.

21. (D) Inability to dorsiflex (evert) the foot or hand indicates a severe nerve dysfunction. This may also be accompanied by loss of sensation or tingling, but these signs are less ominous. Normal capillary refilling should occur in about two seconds. Of course, a strong distal pulse is desirable.

22. (B) A fracture of the maxilla will trap one or more of the muscles controlling eye motion. This is a fracture of the floor of the orbit.

23. (B) The clavicle is considered part of the shoulder girdle.

24. (C) Proper immobilization of a fractured clavicle or scapula can be accomplished by using a sling and swathe. Fractures of these bones can cause severe lung damage. Check breath sounds in these patients for possible pneumothorax. Transport in a position of comfort, usually a sitting position.

25. (C) Shoulder dislocations can be splinted by use of pillows and a sling. Do not attempt to reduce this injury. Distal pulse status is very important. Transport in a sitting position.

26. (A) Applying gentle traction to a fractured humerus will allow for its return to a near normal position. Immobilization can then be accomplished by use of a sling and swathe. Board splints may be used if you are unable to straighten a severely angulated fracture or one that may involve the shoulder joint. Movement of the limb may aid the distal circulation. Traction splints are not used, as they would cause further damage to the nerves and vessels in the axilla.

27. (D) The greatest danger of an elbow injury is that of nerve or vessel damage. Elbow sprains are rarely seen. Injury (fractures, sprains, or dislocations) to the elbow will cause swelling. Epiphyseal fractures are more serious in children, as they may affect growth of the limb.

28. (A) Proper care for a dislocated elbow should include splinting in place when the distal pulse is present. The elbow should not be moved without first contacting your Medical Control for instructions. Generally, one attempt to move the elbow will be authorized, if the distal pulse is absent. This action should be discontinued if resistance or excessive pain is demonstrated.

29. (C) A fracture of the forearm (ulna or radius) should be immobilized at the wrist and elbow. This prevents movement in any plane and may require the use of a sling to immobilize the humerus.

30. (A) An air splint cannot be properly applied to an angulated fracture that should be kept in the position found. Vacuum (bean bag) splints

and rigid splints such as ladders, SAMs, and boards can be adapted to immobilize deformed extremities with little effort.

31. (D) A "Colles fracture" or "silver-fork deformity" involves the radius and ulna. It is often caused by an attempt to break a fall with outstretched arms.

32. (A) Proper care for injuries involving the hands include applying bulky dressings with the hand placed in the position of function. This can be done by placing a roll of roller bandage in the patient's palm and gently closing the fingers around it. The hand can then be elevated to reduce swelling. Dislocated fingers should not be popped back into place by the EMT. The hand can be cooled by ice as long as ice does not come in contact with the skin and the dressings are kept dry.

33. (B) The best management for a severe pelvic fracture is the application of a pneumatic counter-pressure device. The device would effectively immobilize the pelvis and reduce or prevent shock. The patient could then be placed on a spineboard. Second treatment of choice would include application of large cravats and sandbags to help immobilize the pelvis while the patient is on the long spineboard. Traction splints are not indicated.

34. (C) Pelvic fractures are commonly accompanied by severe bleeding into the pelvic cavity and retroperitoneal space. Pelvic fractures are usually closed wounds.

35. (D) Traction splints should not be used on patients found to have dislocated hips. The sciatic nerve lies posterior to the joint; thus, it would be injured in a posterior hip dislocation. Posterior hip dislocation will present with knees drawn up and the affected leg adducted and rotated inward. Abduction and external rotation of the thigh would be observed in an anterior hip dislocation. Anterior dislocations are caused by abduction of the legs. Posterior dislocation is often caused by the knees hitting a dashboard in a MVA.

36. (B) An elderly patient's isolated fracture of the femoral neck can be immobilized by placing the patient on a spineboard and sandbagging or pillow-splinting around the limb. This injury typically presents with the affected leg appearing shorter, with outward rotation. If muscle

spasm is present, a traction splint is indicated. When applied, the torque provided by traction splints should seldom exceed 25 pounds. A pneumatic counter-pressure device should not be inflated in excess of 100 mmHg.

37. (A) A severely injured knee should be splinted in place if a distal pulse is present. Do not attempt to straighten the leg if resistance is felt or patient discomfort increases. Contact your Medical Control for specific instructions. Do not use a traction splint to straighten knee injuries. The device can be used as a basic splint without the use of mechanical traction.

38. (C) Mr. Schubert should have a traction splint applied to his mid-shaft femur fracture. The distal pulse should be palpated before and after splint application. The amount of traction to be applied should generally not exceed 10% of the patient's body weight, or be more than is required to overcome the muscle spasms. The pneumatic counter-pressure device is never applied over a Hare splint. Some splints may be applied outside the PCPD. An air splint is of no value to injuries above the knee.

39. (D) The most frequently fractured bone in the body is the clavicle. Patients with clavicle fractures should be managed with a high degree of suspicion for cervical and head injuries.

40. (C) The patient has jumped from a height sufficient to fracture both of his heels. This force may very well have also injured his spine, often the lumbar area. Application of pillow splints and a long spineboard are indicated. The foot of the spineboard can be elevated to reduce swelling in the feet. Do not exceed an elevation of 12 inches, as this will impair the patient's respirations.

41. (C) The most reliable symptom of a spinal injury is the patient's complaint about pain in the spine. Painful movement is an indicator, along with numbness or tingling. Weakness of one side of the body is also possible, although it is seen more often in head injuries and stroke situations.

42. (C) After the patient has been asked about any pain, tingling, or numbness, a check for deformity can be performed. The patient can then be

asked to move her fingers and toes. If not contraindicated at this point, the patient may attempt gentle movement of the spine to see if pain is produced. Protection of the spine is advised if the mechanism indicates a potential for injury.

43. (A) Generally, the helmet need not be removed in the field if the patient's airway can be adequately maintained. This may require removal of the chin strap or face guard. If the helmet is too large for the patient, it may slip off when the chin strap is cut. A properly fitted helmet must be spread laterally to clear the ears. Full-face helmets must be tipped back to clear the nose. Local policy or Medical Control can assist you in the decision to remove or not remove a helmet in the field.

44. (A) A patient suspected of having cervical spinal injuries should be splinted in the position found if the airway is adequate. His or her position may not facilitate the use of some cervical collars. A rolled sheet may work. Do not release manual traction until the head is completely immobilized. Secure the trunk of the patient to the spineboard before securing the head and neck. Avoid the use of chin straps, as they may compromise the airway.

45. (D) The two most common complications of spinal cord injury are neurogenic shock and paralysis of chest muscles. Observe the patient for chest wall movement and exaggerated abdominal breathing. A high concentration of O_2 is indicated in both cases. Positive-pressure ventilation may also be required.

46. (A) Paresthesia is an abnormal sensation such as numbness, prickling, or tingling. Priapism is an abnormal, painful, and continued erection of the penis. Porphyria is a metabolic disorder that may present as a neurologic disturbance. Peristalsis is the normal wavelike contraction of the intestine.

47. (A) On occasion, a secondary examination may not be performed until life-threatening emergencies are addressed or the patient is loaded for rapid transport to a facility for care of major injuries. A secondary examination is generally considered to include a thorough head-to-toe exam of the body. It is important to start at the head and neck and work down in a systematic manner. The shoulder and thorax should be checked after the head and neck. (The neck may have been already im-

mobilized if a C-spine injury was suspected in the primary exam.) The abdomen should be examined before the pelvis. Repeated use of the same exam procedure will ensure the complete examination of patients who have distracting problems, such as angulated fractures or burns.

48. (C) The humerus should be immobilized at the shoulder and elbow. The most common splinting mistake is failing to immobilize the proximal joint. A humerus can be splinted by use of a sling and swathe or board splints. Evaluate distal neurovascular status.

49. (C) Traction splints should be applied to fractured femurs. A PCPD may be applied to bilateral femur fractures. Traction splints should not be applied to crushed legs, dislocated knees, or ankle fractures.

50. (A) When immobilizing a patient on a backboard, always strap or fix the body trunk before the head. This will ensure a rigid surface for the spine. Manual traction should be maintained until the entire splint is applied. Do not rely on soft cervical collars. Chin straps are generally avoided, as they can lead to two problems if a patient vomits: One, the strap keeps the mouth closed; two, if you release the strap to care for the airway, the head may move around and further injure the spine. Some short boards use straps around the legs of a patient in a sitting position. These straps pull a great deal on the patient's spine when he or she is in the supine position.

51. (B) This is possibly the most controversial answer in this book. Several textbooks instruct you to remove the shoe before application of the traction splint. Some skirt the issue; others say not to remove the shoe. Your Medical Control can best establish local policy for your service, as physicians disagree on this issue. All authorities agree that distal neurovascular status must be checked before and after application of a traction splint. The splints are generally adjusted to length prior to application. This can be done by using the uninjured leg for reference. The ischial straps should be fastened before mechanical traction is applied to keep the splints in proper position. The ankle and lower leg should have traction applied to them to overcome the spasms of the thigh. Protect the dorsal aspect of the foot with adequate padding to avoid tissue damage.

52. (D) Swelling in any restrictive body compartment is dangerous. As swelling occurs, blood vessels are crushed, literally causing a loss of cir-

culation. Nerves are crushed and inadequately perfused; thus, feeling abates. The muscles, also inadequately perfused, begin to die and permanent loss of function is possible. Often called a "compartment syndrome," such an injury is corrected by surgery or treatment in a hyperbaric chamber.

53. (B) Proper care for neurogenic shock includes immobilization on a long spineboard and elevation of the foot of the board. The board should not be elevated more than 12 inches. This height will allow venous return of pooled blood in the lower extremities without significant shift of the abdominal contents. Should the bowels shift, undue pressure may be exerted on the diaphragm leading to increasing difficulty in breathing.

54. (B) Injury to the peroneal nerve, found behind the knee and lateral just below the knee, will cause the patient to lose the ability to dorsiflex the foot. A dropped foot is typical. Sensation will also be lost in the great toe and on the lateral side of the foot. The toes may still be able to "grip" but will be unable to dorsiflex or evert. Rigid splints applied over the peroneal nerve must be well padded to prevent nerve complications.

55. (D) When the patellas are on the same plane bilaterally, you can generally rule out injury above the knee, unless, of course, there are bilateral injuries proximally.

56. (A) Patients with pelvic fractures often have blood losses between 1000 cc and 3000 cc. Of course, this amount of blood loss can lead to profound shock, even death. Patients with femoral fractures involving the shaft often lose between 500 cc and 1000 cc of blood. Patients with fractures of the radius/ulna may lose between 250 cc and 500 cc of blood, while tibia/fibula fracture may result in slightly more than a 250–600 cc blood loss. These figures are for closed fractures.

57. (B) The EMT can differentiate a pelvic fracture from a hip fracture by pelvic compression. Apply pressure on the iliac crests. If pain is present, the pelvis is unstable. Both hip and pelvic injuries can cause an inability to move the leg, high leg pain, and crepitus (grating sounds).

8 Nervous System and Head Injuries

The nervous system, spine, and head injuries are addressed in Chapter 8. The EMT must be able to manage injuries to the head, neck, and spine so that there is minimal risk of a potentially disabling injury to the patient. Questions are included on the proper assessment of a spine or head injury, the possible complications that may result from such an injury, and immobilization techniques.

Several questions relate to proper emergency care for injuries to the eyes, as well as to the face and skull. Common injuries discussed include whiplash, concussion, avulsed scalp, and crush injuries to the airway. The Glascow Coma Scale is also reviewed in this chapter.

1. Acting as a control center for respiration, one of the most primitive parts of the brain is the:

   A. Cerebrum.
   B. Cerebellum.
   C. Thalamus.
   D. Medulla oblongata.

2. Body movement of the left side of the body is controlled by which portion of the brain?

   A. Front.
   B. Rear.
   C. Right.
   D. Left.

3. The nervous system that regulates voluntary muscle function is the:

   A. Autonomic nervous system.
   B. Involuntary nervous system.
   C. Parasympathetic nervous system.
   D. Somatic nervous system.

4. The meninges are a set of coverings that suspends and protects the brain and spinal cord. Choose the correct statement regarding the components of the meninges.

   A. The dura mater is a filmy layer.
   B. The cerebrospinal fluid (CSF) is between the arachnoid and pia mater.
   C. The pia mater lies between the dura mater and the arachnoid layer.
   D. The blood vessels nourishing the brain run in the dura mater.

5. The sympathetic nervous system lies parallel to and outside of the spinal canal. It is responsible for:

   A. Increases in heart rate, relaxation of sphincters, and dilation of blood vessels.
   B. Increases in heart rate, constriction of sphincters, and dilation of blood vessels.
   C. Decreases in heart rate, constriction of sphincters, and dilation of blood vessels.

D. Increases in heart rate, constriction of sphincters, and constriction of blood vessels.

6. The spinal cord ends as a single structure and creates the configuration called the cauda equina (horsetail) at vertebra number:

    A. Thoracic 12.
    B. Lumbar 2.
    C. Cervical 7.
    D. Sacral 4.

7. A concussion is best described as an injury:

    A. Caused by closed deceleration of the brain.
    B. Causing minor bleeding within the skull.
    C. Judged to be less severe if retrograde amnesia is present.
    D. That always renders the patient unconscious for a period of time.

8. The most important neurological observation you can make when charting the status of a patient with a head injury is his or her:

    A. Response to pain stimuli.
    B. Pupillary reaction to light.
    C. Change in the level of consciousness.
    D. Vital signs.

9. Nearly 70% of the unrestrained people involved in motor vehicle accidents sustain injuries to the skull and brain. Choose the most appropriate statement about unconscious patients with head injuries.

    A. Cyanosis is almost always present.
    B. Breathing will almost always be slow and shallow.
    C. An unconscious head injury patient should not be turned on the side.
    D. Cervical injuries should be suspected in all of these patients.

10. Profuse bleeding from scalp injuries is very common. Choose the correct statement about the scalp.

    A. The surface layer of the scalp is thin and the underlying tissue (galea aponeurotica) is extremely thick.
    B. Bleeding from the scalp is usually controlled by direct pressure.

C. Scalp wounds that are wide open or avulsed should be bandaged in the position found.
D. Direct local pressure should be applied to all scalp wounds, regardless of other injuries.

11. A thorough exam of a patient with suspected spinal injuries may give a clue to the location of the spinal lesion or fracture. From the following statements, select the correct one.

    A. Heavy abdominal breathing and little chest movement indicate a lesion around C5 C6.
    B. Reaction produced by pin-pricking at nipple level indicates injury at T10.
    C. A loss of sensation in the arms indicates a lesion above C3.
    D. A loss of sensation in the legs indicates a lesion below S2.

12. A patient who is bleeding within the skull and has no other injuries will most likely produce which of the following sets of vitals?

    A. Lowering blood pressure, slowing pulse, and increasing respiratory rate.
    B. Lowering blood pressure, slowing pulse, and decreasing respiratory rate.
    C. Rising blood pressure, rising pulse, and decreasing respiratory rate.
    D. Rising blood pressure, slowing pulse, and decreasing respiratory rate.

13. The type of response noted when a patient reacts to pain stimuli but is ineffective in protecting him or her would receive a partial Glascow Coma score of:

    A. 1.
    B. 2.
    C. 3.
    D. 4.

14. A patient who gives inappropriate verbal responses to questions would receive a partial Glascow Coma score of:

    A. 5.
    B. 4.

C. 3.
D. 2.

15. A patient who only opens his eyes upon painful stimuli would receive a partial Glascow Coma score of:

    A. 4.
    B. 3.
    C. 2.
    D. 1.

16. The least ominous pupillary sign in a patient with head injuries is pupils that are of:

    A. Equal size and do not constrict.
    B. Unequal size and constrict in response to light.
    C. Unequal size and one constricts, one remains fixed.
    D. Equal size and constrict with bright light.

17. A clear, watery fluid is escaping from the right ear of an unconscious MVA patient. There is also ecchymosis under the eyes. You should:

    A. Apply ice packs to the eyes and pack the ear.
    B. Apply ice packs to the eyes and ear.
    C. Cover both eyes with moist dressings and pressure-dress the ear.
    D. Make no attempt to control the escape of fluid from the ears.

18. The most important care an EMT can provide the patient with a foreign object impaled in the skull is to:

    A. Control bleeding from the edges of the wound.
    B. Cover open wounds properly.
    C. Splint the cervical spine.
    D. Maintain an open airway.

19. Proper care for a patient with head injuries includes:

    A. Positioning the patient with the head slightly down.
    B. Placing the head on a pillow on a level stretcher.
    C. Administering supplemental O_2.
    D. Suctioning of the patient's airway every 10–15 seconds.

20. A 43-year-old female has fallen down a flight of stairs. She is having a seizure when you arrive. There is evidence of a pinkish fluid coming from her ears and nose. After about one minute, her seizure ceases. Further exam reveals a closed fracture of the left tibia. You should:

    A. Transport her immediately.
    B. Immobilize her neck and transport.
    C. Immobilize her tibia and transport.
    D. Immobilize her spine and leg, then transport.

21. Probably the most rapidly progressive hematoma to occur within the cranium is a/an:

    A. Subdural hematoma.
    B. Epidural hematoma.
    C. Intracerebral hematoma.
    D. Intracranial hematoma.

22. Frequently, a patient will refuse transportation even though you may suspect a minor head injury. The patient should be instructed to watch, or to be watched, for certain signs or symptoms of a head injury. Among these signs are confusion or disorientation and:

    A. Lowering body temperature.
    B. Nausea or vomiting.
    C. Intermittent headaches.
    D. Rising pulse rate.

23. The clear, jellylike fluid that maintains the shape of the eye is the:

    A. Aqueous humor.
    B. Vitreous humor.
    C. Conjunctiva.
    D. Choroid.

24. Made up of tough, fibrous tissue, the white part of the eye is the:

    A. Cornea.
    B. Iris.
    C. Retina.
    D. Sclera.

25. Choose the correct statement regarding foreign bodies on or in the eye.

   A. Foreign bodies under the upper eyelid or on the cornea can easily be removed by irrigation.
   B. To prevent further injury, large impaled foreign bodies should be removed before transportation.
   C. Only the injured eye should be covered.
   D. Many foreign bodies can be washed out by irrigation with saline or eye irrigation solutions.

26. Chemical burns to the eye are commonly caused by acids and alkalis. Choose the appropriate care for such an injury.

   A. Alkali burns should be irrigated for at least 20 minutes.
   B. Acid burns should be irrigated for at least 20 minutes.
   C. Only sterile saline solution should be used on eye injuries.
   D. The eyelids should never be forced open during irrigation, as closing them is a natural protective reflex.

27. The following statements deal with thermal and light burns to the eye. The correct statement is:

   A. When a face is exposed to fire, the eyeballs are frequently burned.
   B. Light burns from an arc welder are extremely painful immediately after exposure.
   C. Exposure to infrared rays causes injury to the lens and is seldom permanent.
   D. "Snow blindness" may produce extreme pain three to five hours after exposure.

28. A 22-year-old female presents with a laceration of her right upper eyelid. Profuse bleeding hinders your exam of the eyeball itself. After the bleeding stops, you should:

   A. Cover both eyes to decrease movement.
   B. Use heavy direct pressure on the eye and lid to control bleeding.
   C. Cover both eyes with protective cups.
   D. Apply dry, sterile dressings directly to her right eye after the bleeding is controlled.

29. General guidelines for unconscious patients with soft contact lenses include:

   A. Noting presence of lenses on chart but making no attempt to remove them in the field.
   B. Removal if eye injury is obvious.
   C. Removal of a soft lens by pinching it off the eye.
   D. Leaving the eyes open and untaped, as they will not dry with lenses in place.

30. Which of the following reflects proper care for a patient with head injuries?

   A. Objects penetrating the cheek should not be removed in the field.
   B. A patient with a severe head injury and signs of shock should only be transported with the head down and legs elevated.
   C. An avulsed scalp should be washed and replaced in its normal position.
   D. A patient with extreme facial fractures and hemorrhage should not be suctioned, as it will dislodge clots and increase bleeding.

31. A 20-year-old female has fallen while blade-skating and struck her unprotected head. You would anticipate that she may vomit and:

   A. Experience convulsions.
   B. Have a rapid fall in blood pressure.
   C. Have a rapid rise in pulse rate.
   D. Have pinpoint pupils.

32. A patient with a brain contusion would most likely show signs of:

   A. Progressively improved neurological activity.
   B. Dilation of both pupils.
   C. Paralysis on one side of the body.
   D. Falling blood pressure.

33. A patient with severe bleeding from large vessels about the neck must be protected from air embolism by:

   A. Sitting the patient up.
   B. Applying direct pressure to the vessels at the laceration.

C. Applying direct pressure to the artery below the laceration.
D. Applying direct pressure to the vessels above and below the laceration.

34. What should you do with teeth that have become dislodged due to trauma?

    A. Place the teeth in ice water.
    B. Wrap the teeth in dry, sterile dressings.
    C. Maintain the teeth in a warm, moist environment.
    D. Do nothing since teeth cannot be reimplanted.

35. You are treating a patient who has received facial injuries in a barroom altercation. Your initial examination reveals only some swelling and local pain. Select the best clue of possible facial fractures.

    A. Dry mouth.
    B. Bruised lips.
    C. Bloody nose.
    D. Irregular bite.

Answers with Rationale

1. (D) The medulla oblongata controls respirations and is located in the lowermost area of the brain. The cerebellum fine-tunes movement, is located below the great mass of cerebral tissue, and is known as the little brain.

2. (C) The right side of the brain controls the left side of the body. The front part of the brain controls emotions. Speech is controlled deep within the brain.

3. (D) The somatic nervous system regulates the function of voluntary muscles. The involuntary nervous system is also known as the autonomic nervous system.

4. (B) The CSF is between the filmy layers of the arachnoid and pia mater. The dura mater is the tough, leatherlike layer next to the skull. Blood vessels nourishing the brain run in the arachnoid and pia mater.

5. (D) The sympathetic nervous system is responsible for increases in heart rate, constriction of the sphincters, and constriction of blood vessels. The para-sympathetic nervous system's function is the opposite of the sympathetic, involving decreases in heart rate, relaxation of the sphincters, and dilation of blood vessels.

6. (B) The spinal cord ends as a single structure at L2. From that point on, the nerve bundles are broken down into smaller structures.

7. (A) Concussions are generally caused by deceleration of the brain against the skull. The patient may be only stunned, not always rendered unconscious. The greater the degree of amnesia (retrograde—cannot remember events prior to injury), the greater the severity of the injury. Ask the patient what he or she remembers last, before the accident occurred, and record the response verbatim in the patient's medical records. There isn't any bleeding within the skull unless it is contused.

8. (C) The lowering level of consciousness (LOC) is always the best indicator of progressive head injury. LOC includes response to verbal or pain stimuli, pupillary response, respiratory effort, and motor move-

ment. The introduction of painful stimuli is another check of the LOC. Vital signs may be deceptive, as in the case of shock and head injury. Pupil reaction will be affected later, as the patient's condition worsens.

9. (D) Cervical injuries should be suspected in all unconscious patients with head injuries. Cyanosis is seldom caused by head injury alone. Breathing patterns will usually be deep, often irregular. The patient is best transported with the head turned (whole body if on spineboard) to allow for drainage of secretions.

10. (B) Profuse bleeding from the scalp is most often controlled by heavy direct pressure unless there is suspicion of underlying skull fracture. The scalp has two layers: the outer, which is very thick on the surface, and the thin, extremely strong fascial tissue or galea. Open scalp wounds should be closed and pressure exerted on them to control bleeding.

11. (A) Heavy abdominal breathing and little chest movement indicate a lesion in the area of C5 C6. Pain stimuli felt at nipple level indicates a lesion around T4. The arms generally relate to C4 through T1. The legs are generally connected by nerves branching out above S2.

12. (D) A patient with a head injury usually exhibits a rise in blood pressure, slowing pulse rate, and slowing and/or irregular respiratory rate.

13. (D) A response to pain stimuli that is ineffective in protecting the patient is said to be inappropriate and would receive a partial Glascow Coma score of 4. If a decerebrate response (extension or stiffening upon the introduction of pain) is noted, a Glascow score of 2 is awarded. A decorticate response that demonstrates extension of the lower extremities and the arms in flexion receives a 3. A patient who does not respond to pain receives a 1.

14. (C) A patient who gives inappropriate verbal responses to questions would get a partial Glascow Coma score of 3. An oriented response receives a 5. Confused verbal responses are given a 4; incomprehensible response, 2. No response is a 1.

15. (C) Spontaneous eye opening receives a partial Glascow Coma score of 4. Eye opening to voice command, 3. To pain, 2. No eye opening by the patient receives a score of 1.

16. (D) The least ominous pupillary sign would be equal pupils that constrict to pinpoint when a bright light is shone into them. Any negative change of pupil size or responsiveness indicates progressive brain damage in head injury.

17. (D) Make no attempt to control the escape of CSF from the ears or nose. Any control might increase intracranial pressures and provide a "wick" for infection to be introduced to the brain. Ice can be applied to the eyes to reduce swelling. There is no need to reduce eye movement, but it should be observed for equality.

18. (D) Airway maintenance is always the most important care an EMT can render. Foreign objects impaled in the skull should be covered with moist dressings to prevent drying of tissue. Bleeding should be controlled at the edges of the wound, but deep bleeding should not be hindered. Splint the spine, as it may very well be unstable.

19. (C) A patient with a head injury should have O_2 administered to reduce swelling of the brain. Once the patient's spine is immobilized, the patient's head can be slightly elevated. Particular caution must be paid to the C-spine, as many patients with head trauma have concurrent C-spine injury. Suctioning should be used only as needed because it tends to increase intracranial pressure.

20. (D) Even though this patient has a severe head injury, her other problems must be addressed before she is transported. A cervical injury must be suspected and immobilized and her fractured tibia should also be splinted prior to transportation unless directed to do otherwise by your Medical Control.

21. (B) All of the distractors listed are intracranial hematomas. An epidural hematoma occurs when blood flows between the dura and the cranial bones. Since most of this bleeding is arterial, a true emergency exists. A subdural hematoma is caused by bleeding between the meninges and the brain and is usually slow venous flow. An intracerebral hematoma can occur spontaneously in patients with high blood pressure, causing a stroke.

22. (B) Nausea and vomiting often accompany head injuries. Body temperature usually rises in a patient with a head injury. Headaches will be persistent and the pulse rate may fall.

23. (B) The vitreous humor is the clear, jellylike fluid found in the posterior chamber of the eye. The aqueous humor is watery and located in the anterior chamber between the lens and cornea. The choroid is a layer of blood vessels between the retina and sclera. The conjunctiva is a smooth mucous membrane covering the sclera and inside of the eyelids.

24. (D) The sclera is the white of the eye. The clear, transparent tissue over the opening of the eye is the cornea. The muscle that regulates pupil size is the iris, the tissue that gives the eye its characteristic color. The retina is the light-sensitive layer in the back of the eye.

25. (D) Many foreign bodies can be irrigated out of the eye by working with the head tilted so that the solution flows from medial to lateral. Foreign bodies under the upper lid or on the cornea are difficult to remove by irrigation. The upper eyelid may be everted. The cornea should not be touched. Foreign bodies impaling the eye should never be removed in the field. Both the eyes, injured and uninjured, should be covered, as they tend to track one another, causing further damage to the injured eye.

26. (A) Alkali burns should be irrigated for at least 20 minutes. Sterile saline solution or eye wash is preferred, but plain water may be used. Eyelids may require forceful opening to facilitate proper irrigation. Aggressive management in the field may prevent permanent damage to the patient. Acid burns are treated by flushing with water for at least 5 minutes.

27. (D) "Snow blindness" or exposure to ultraviolet rays may cause extreme pain of the eyes hours after exposure, as the cornea begins to break down. Light burns from an arc welder are similar to that of snow blindness. Infrared rays burn the retina and are generally not painful; however, permanent visual damage may occur. The eyeballs themselves are seldom burned in a fire, as the lids quickly close to protect them.

28. (A) Covering both eyes will reduce movement that may dislodge clots. Heavy direct pressure should not be used on the eyeball itself, especially if there is a laceration of the eyeball. Dry dressings should not come in contact with the eye. The dressings should first be moistened with saline or other sterile solutions.

29. (C) A soft lens may be removed by pinching it off the eye. A contact lens should not be removed if an eye injury is evident. An eye will dry rapidly, even with a lens in, so remove lens if possible, close the lid, and either tape the eye shut or place moist dressings over both eyes.

30. (C) An avulsed scalp can be washed off and replaced in its normal position to reduce bleeding and preserve the tissue. Penetrating objects in the cheek often must be removed to control hemorrhaging. A patient with severe head injury and shock can be transported with the legs elevated and head slightly elevated. The patient with massive facial fractures and hemorrhage will need to be suctioned frequently or blood clots may occlude the airway.

31. (A) A patient with a head injury may vomit and experience convulsions. Some head injury patients become very violent and must be restrained. Keep in mind that their violence, although perhaps directed at you, is part of their injury. Protect yourself but don't become angered by the patient's behavior. A violent patient can be restrained by sandwiching them face-down (prone) between the stretcher mattress and a scoop stretcher if not contraindicated by other injuries.

32. (C) A brain contusion may produce signs of paralysis on one side of the body or sometimes of the lower extremities. The neurological signs will progressively deteriorate, and the blood pressure will rise. Generally, only one pupil will be affected until late in the process.

33. (D) Direct pressure to vessels above and below the point of a laceration will reduce the chance of air embolism. The patient should be kept in a head-down position.

34. (C) Dislodged teeth should be kept warm and moist. One possible location is in the patient's mouth if he or she is conscious and able to adequately control the airway and gag reflex.

35 (D) An irregular bite, increased salivation, bleeding in the mouth, and inability to swallow or talk are all clues of possible facial fractures. Any patient with a significant facial fracture is at risk of developing an airway obstruction. Constant monitoring of the airway for bleeding or swelling is indicated in such a patient.

9 Chest, Abdominal, and Genital Injuries

A great deal of information is included in the rationale regarding injuries to the chest and the correct treatment for these often life-threatening conditions. Thorough understanding of the potential progression of a chest injury may help you to save many severely injured patients during your career.

Complaints involving the abdomen are voiced by patients regularly. Understanding the anatomy and physiology of organs located within the abdomen may help you determine the severity of the patient's problem, the immediate care required, and the speed of transportation appropriate to the malady.

Also discussed are injuries to the urinary bladder, female reproductive organs, and the more often injured male genitalia. The EMT will be summoned to care for patients with problems ranging from unexplained stomach pains to open wounds of the abdomen. Correct treatment, such as proper positioning of the patient, can do much to relieve pain and reduce morbidity and mortality.

1. The proper order of care for a patient with chest injuries is to first open and maintain the airway and then to:

   A. Administer supplemental O_2.
   B. Record vital signs.
   C. Control obvious external bleeding.
   D. Observe for any respiratory change.

2. The best way to care for a patient with fractured ribs is by:

   A. Placing him or her on the uninjured side.
   B. Applying adhesive tape around the chest wall.
   C. Applying a sling and swath over the area of the fracture.
   D. Doing nothing to restrict chest wall movement.

3. Signs of significant chest injury include:

   A. Pain at the site of injury and expansion of both sides of the chest on inhalation.
   B. Hemoptysis and dyspnea.
   C. Cyanosis of the lips and weak pulse.
   D. Expansion of both sides of the chest on inhalation and low blood pressure.

4. The ribs that are most often fractured are the:

   A. Upper 4.
   B. 5th through 9th.
   C. 11th and 12th.
   D. 13th and 14th.

5. A patient's upper body appears cyanotic, and the neck veins and eyes bulge. Which type of chest injury should you suspect?

   A. Pneumothorax.
   B. Hemothorax.
   C. Subcutaneous emphysema.
   D. Traumatic asphyxia.

6. A patient with a flail chest often has paradoxical motion of the chest wall (segments moving in the opposite direction of normal respiratory movement). Dangers involved in this type of injury include:

   A. Overexpansion of the lungs.

B. Contusion of the underlying lung.
C. Excess uptake of O_2.
D. Excess blowing off of CO_2.

7. The most important care you can give a cyanotic patient with a flail chest is:

    A. Sandbagging of the sternum.
    B. Pillow splinting of the flail segment.
    C. Artificial ventilation.
    D. Supplemental O_2.

8. The term that best describes the condition in which increasing amounts of air become trapped in the pleural space during each breath is:

    A. Tension pneumothorax.
    B. Spontaneous pneumothorax.
    C. Pneumothorax.
    D. Subcutaneous emphysema.

9. What should you do for a patient with a penetrating chest injury who develops signs of a tension pneumothorax?

    A. Transport the patient on his or her injured side.
    B. Release the occlusive chest dressing.
    C. Transport the patient on his or her uninjured side.
    D. Suction the patient's airway to relieve the tension.

10. Signs of tension pneumothorax include:

    A. A rise in blood pressure, cyanosis.
    B. A strong, bounding pulse with distended neck veins.
    C. Bulging neck veins, increasing respiratory difficulty.
    D. Flattened neck veins, low blood pressure.

11. Your first priority of care for a patient with a sucking chest wound is to:

    A. Administer O_2.
    B. Seal the wound.
    C. Examine for exit wounds.
    D. Listen for breath sounds over the injured lung.

12. Choose the best statement regarding pulmonary contusion.

    A. A pulmonary contusion will always cause respiratory distress.
    B. A pulmonary contusion never develops signs in less than 48 hours.
    C. Care for a patient with a pulmonary contusion will require administration of O_2.
    D. A pulmonary contusion has nothing to do with the blood vessels of the lungs.

13. Pericardial tamponade is a condition best described as:

    A. Fluid in the lung space.
    B. Fluid in the sac surrounding the heart.
    C. Crepitus under the skin.
    D. A condition present with hemothorax.

14. When performing artificial ventilation on a patient with a sealed, sucking chest wound, it is important to:

    A. Use smaller ventilations than normal.
    B. Open the occlusive dressing on the wound.
    C. Keep the patient on the injured side.
    D. Not allow your ventilations to cause chest rise.

15. Mr. Barnes has been involved in a serious head-on MVA. He is unconscious and has distended neck veins, difficulty in breathing, and a weak pulse. The last three blood pressure readings have been 110/70, 100/80, and 96/86, respectively. You should suspect that Mr. Barnes' life-threatening problem is a:

    A. Pulmonary contusion.
    B. Myocardial infarction.
    C. Hemothorax.
    D. Pericardial tamponade.

16. Which of the following organs is located in the retroperitoneal space?

    A. Spleen.
    B. Pancreas.
    C. Liver.
    D. Bile ducts.

17. From the choices below, select the answer that lists only hollow organs.

    A. Liver, spleen, stomach, and gallbladder.
    B. Stomach, gallbladder, bile ducts, and kidneys.
    C. Gallbladder, small intestine, pancreas, and appendix.
    D. Stomach, bile ducts, urinary bladder, and appendix.

18. The smooth, thin, glistening layer of transparent tissue lining the abdomen is the:

    A. Pleura.
    B. Serosa.
    C. Peritoneum.
    D. Mesentery.

19. The hormone produced in the pancreas that regulates the amount of sugar in the blood is:

    A. Pepsin.
    B. Insulin.
    C. Ptyalin.
    D. Bile.

20. The coordinated, wavelike contraction of the gastrointestinal tract is called:

    A. Pleurisy.
    B. Peritonitis.
    C. Peristalsis.
    D. Pyelonephritis.

21. The first part of the small intestine is the:

    A. Duodenum.
    B. Jejunum.
    C. Ileum.
    D. Cecum.

22. The abdominal mesentery can be torn or lacerated during high-speed deceleration. Choose the correct statement regarding such an injury.

    A. A tear of the mesentery can produce peritonitis by spilling its contents into the abdomen.

B. Bleeding from a tear of the mesentery is seldom severe.
C. A tear of the mesentery may cause a loss of blood supply to the organ to which it is connected.
D. A tear of the mesentery seldom causes abdominal distention.

23. Choose the correct statement regarding closed abdominal injuries.

    A. Blood within the peritoneal cavity is extremely irritating.
    B. Little pain will result from bowel contents being released into the peritoneal cavity.
    C. Injuries involving the descending aorta or venae cavae could be considered abdominal injuries.
    D. Muscle rigidity, intense pain, and tenderness is seen only in solid-organ injuries of the abdomen.

24. Upon your arrival at an unknown illness call, you find a 53-year-old man, Mr. Kocker, lying on his right side with his legs drawn up. He complains of severe pains in his belly. After loosening his clothing, your next action should be to:

    A. Palpate his abdomen.
    B. Straighten his legs.
    C. Record vital signs.
    D. Administer instant glucose.

25. Mr. Kocker may be positioned on his back if he finds it more comfortable. Your examination reveals abdominal tenderness and rigidity. You would expect his respirations to be:

    A. Slow and deep.
    B. Slow and shallow.
    C. Rapid and deep.
    D. Rapid and shallow.

26. During your visual exam of the abdomen, you notice a halfmoon-shaped bruise under Mr. Kocker's costal arch. You would suspect:

    A. Little relationship between the bruise and abdominal pain.
    B. Abdominal trauma at least two months earlier.
    C. Abdominal trauma 12–24 hours earlier.
    D. Acute appendicitis.

27. Proper care for an evisceration should include applying:

    A. Ice to reduce swelling.
    B. Moist, sterile dressings and aluminum foil.
    C. Dry, sterile dressings to provide a matrix for clotting.
    D. Moist, sterile dressings with ice packs.

28. Choose the correct statement regarding characteristics and symptoms of abdominal injuries.

    A. Peritonitis will be more rapidly caused by blood in the peritoneal cavity than by bowel contents.
    B. Solid-organ injuries usually release digested and undigested food into the peritoneal cavity.
    C. Foreign objects impaled in the abdomen should be removed in the field to facilitate control of bleeding.
    D. Pulsing or throbbing masses felt during the abdominal exam indicate a need for rapid transportation.

29. Select the correct statement regarding the parietal and visceral peritoneum.

    A. The visceral peritoneum is the lining of the wall of the abdomen and perceives sensations similar to those felt by the skin.
    B. The visceral peritoneum sensory nerves are better able to localize an irritating point than the parietal nerves.
    C. Referred pain arises from the visceral peritoneum and its autonomic nervous system.
    D. The parietal peritoneum can only perceive pain caused by stretching or distention of the abdomen.

30. In the United States, the disease most commonly associated with hematemesis is:

    A. Esophageal varices.
    B. Gastritis.
    C. Peptic ulcer.
    D. Dysphagia.

31. Select the correct statement regarding an acute abdomen.

    A. Peritonitis is always associated with a loss of body fluid and may lead to shock.

B. Patients with peritonitis seldom vomit since there is paralysis of normal intestinal peristalsis (ileus).
C. High fevers are generally evident 12–20 hours before an appendix rupture.
D. Abdominal palpation should be vigorous to assure all underlying organs are felt.

32. Proper prehospital care for an acute abdomen includes administration of:

    A. Warm water to break up gas.
    B. 10 grains of aspirin to relieve pain.
    C. Ice packs to reduce distention.
    D. O_2 as a precaution for shock.

33. What disease should you suspect in an acute abdomen patient with localized pain in the back and lower right quadrant?

    A. Appendicitis.
    B. Aortic aneurysm (dissected or ruptured).
    C. Pancreatitis.
    D. Duodenal ulcer.

34. Generalized pain in an acute abdomen would lead you to suspect:

    A. Perforated peptic ulcer.
    B. Cholecystitis.
    C. Diverticulitis.
    D. Kidney stones.

35. A typical source of pain in the lower left quadrant of the abdomen is:

    A. Gastritis.
    B. Intestinal obstruction.
    C. Pancreatitis.
    D. Myocardial ischemia.

36. In which abdominal quadrant would hepatitis present pain?

    A. Upper left.
    B. Upper right.
    C. Lower left.
    D. Lower right.

37. Select the most appropriate response with regard to blunt abdominal wounds.

    A. An empty urinary bladder is more likely to rupture in a rapid deceleration than one which is distended.
    B. Properly worn combination lap/shoulder safety belts seldom cause injury to victims.
    C. The liver and spleen are often lacerated by lap belts worn above the iliac crests of the pelvis.
    D. A patient with isolated blunt abdominal trauma can be transported in a supine position.

38. Within the urinary system, two kidneys produce about 1.5–2.0 liters of urine a day. In a female, urine is passed to a reservoir through a tube known as the:

    A. Uterus.
    B. Urethra.
    C. Ureter.
    D. Bladder.

39. Select the following sign, symptom, or complaint you would most likely find in a patient experiencing renal colic or "passing stones."

    A. Elevated blood pressure.
    B. Localized abdominal pain.
    C. Slowed pulse rate.
    D. Dry skin.

40. A woman of childbearing age may have an unknown ectopic pregnancy that could lead to an acute abdomen. Your care for this patient should include:

    A. Hot packs on the belly.
    B. Soliciting menstrual cycle history.
    C. Transportation on her right side.
    D. Transportation on her stomach.

41. Which of the following statements reflects the correct care of a sexually assaulted adult woman?

    A. Assist the patient in douching before transporting.

B. Unless bleeding is obvious, a female EMT should perform a thorough exam of the genitalia.
C. Transport the patient using your emergency signaling devices (red lights and siren).
D. Cease care if the patient refuses or withdraws consent even though a felony has probably been committed.

42. You are called to an industrial accident and find Mr. Johnson lying on the ground, curled into a ball, bleeding profusely from his genitalia. His penis has been traumatically amputated by a machine. Your immediate care for Mr. Johnson will be:

    A. Direct pressure to control bleeding.
    B. Application of dry, sterile dressings.
    C. Transportation of the amputated penile shaft in moist dressings.
    D. Application of a tourniquet around the remaining stump.

43. Choose the correct statement regarding genitourinary injuries.

    A. Kidney damage is seen only in patients with fractured ribs or penetrating wounds.
    B. Urinary bladder tears are seen only with pelvic fractures.
    C. Pelvic fractures seldom injure internal female genitalia.
    D. Heavy vaginal bleeding may be controlled by packing the vagina.

Answers with Rationale

1. **(A)** Supplemental O_2 should be given to a chest injury patient as soon as possible. Injuries may have already compromised the ability to properly oxygenate the blood because of the presence of blood in the lungs, reduced respiratory movement, or air in the pleural spaces. Next, obvious bleeding should be controlled. Vital signs should then be taken and the patient constantly observed for any change in respiratory status.

2. **(C)** A sling and swath over an area of fractured ribs will do much to reduce the pain experienced while breathing but will still allow some needed chest movement. Circumferential taping of the chest will reduce the ability of the chest to expand and, although the patient seems more comfortable, will be detrimental to the patient. The patient may be transported on the injured side.

3. **(B)** Hemoptysis (coughing up of red blood) and dyspnea (labored breathing) are excellent indicators of significant chest or lung injury. The chest should be observed for equal rise of both sides and palpated for tenderness. A patient with severe chest injuries may produce signs similar to shock and, in fact, may very well be in shock.

4. **(B)** The 5th through 9th ribs are most often fractured. The 4 upper ribs are less susceptible to fractures, as they are protected by more muscle mass. The 11th and 12th float ribs are attached only at the vertebral spine.

5. **(D)** A chest injury patient with bulging eyes and neck veins and profound cyanosis of the upper body has most likely had his or her chest crushed circumferentially. The patient would be said to have experienced traumatic asphyxia. A patient with a hemothorax will have diminished breath sounds on the injured side.

6. **(B)** Contusion of the underlying lung is often much more severe than one might suspect in a flail chest. Much effort is needed to cause the paradoxical motion of the flail segment, and lung bruising occurs easily. Although much respiratory effort takes place, the exchange of gases is greatly reduced.

7. (C) Although immobilization of a flail segment is important, artificial ventilation should be started if the patient exhibits signs of cyanosis. The cyanosis indicates inadequate perfusion and hypoxia in the patient. High-concentration O_2 will also be beneficial.

8. (A) If increasing amounts of air become trapped in the pleural space in either an open or closed chest injury, a tension pneumothorax will occur. This pressure will continue to increase, collapsing the lung on the injured side, bulging intercostal tissue, and causing a shift of the mediastinum, which in turn affects the other hemithorax. The patient's trachea will shift away from the injured side and the injured hemithorax will sound hyperresonant (hollow) if a tension pneumothorax is present. This is a true life-threatening emergency and must be relieved as soon as possible. Pneumothorax is the presence of air within the chest cavity outside of the lung.

9. (B) Should a tension pneumothorax develop in a patient with an open chest wound, simply releasing the occlusive dressing over the wound during exhalation should benefit the patient greatly. You may choose to transport the patient on the injured side, unless contraindicated by other injuries.

10. (C) The neck veins will become distended as venous return is reduced by the pressure on the great vessels. There will be increasing respiratory difficulty and cyanosis as the blood pressure begins to fall. The pulse becomes weaker as the heart also is compressed by the air in the pleural space.

11. (B) Sucking chest wounds should be sealed as soon as they are identified. If you're not sure that it is sucking, seal it anyway. Then administer high-concentration O_2 and examine the chest thoroughly for any other wounds. Listening for breath sounds over each lung field may be done after the other actions are completed.

12. (C) A patient with a pulmonary contusion (bruise to the lungs and blood vessels within) will require supplemental O_2. There is a probability of blood (hemothorax) in the lungs, reducing the surface area of alveoli available for gas exchange. A pulmonary contusion may not demonstrate signs for up to 48 hours after injury. Respiratory distress is not always noted, depending on the severity of the contusion.

13. **(B)** Pericardial (peri = around/cardia = heart) tamponade (tampon = plug) is blood or fluid in the pericardium (nonexpandable sac around the heart), which fills and actually crushes the heart. Blood can no longer fill the chambers of the heart, and circulation is reduced to a point that may cause death. Crepitus is often noted under the skin of patients suffering traumatic asphyxia.

14. **(B)** When performing artificial ventilation on a patient with a sealed, sucking chest wound, it is important to release the occlusive dressing to allow the excess air in the pleural space to escape. Positive pressure from your mouth or other device will expand the lungs and adequately ventilate the patient. Normal chest rise should be observed.

15. **(D)** Pericardial tamponade presents with narrowing pulse pressure readings (systolic and diastolic coming closer together). This is caused by the pericardium filling with blood and not allowing complete filling of the heart. The pulse will also be very weak and heart sounds will become more difficult to hear. Neck veins may also be distended due to high venous pressure. This is a true medical emergency and should be transported rapidly to the Emergency Department. Early radio contact with the hospital may do much to save this patient's life. You may be directed to apply the PCPD to "overperfuse" the heart, stretching the myocardial muscle, which will, upon contraction, produce a greater cardiac output.

16. **(B)** The pancreas is located in the retroperitoneal space, along with the kidneys, ureters, adrenal glands, and much of the duodenum. The spleen, liver, and bile ducts are in the upper quadrants of the abdominal cavity.

17. **(D)** The hollow organs of the abdomen include the stomach, duodenum, small and large intestines, gallbladder, appendix, bile ducts, ureters, and bladder. The solid organs of the abdomen include the liver, spleen, pancreas, adrenal glands, and kidneys.

18. **(C)** The peritoneum is the smooth, thin, glistening lining of the abdomen. The pleura is the lining of the thorax. The serosa is the covering of the abdominal organs made up of peritoneum. The mesentery is a peritoneal fold connecting the intestine to the posterior abdominal wall.

19. **(B)** Insulin is a hormone produced in the pancreas, more specifically in the "islets of Langerhans." Pepsin is a digestive enzyme found in the stomach. Ptyalin is a digestive enzyme found in the saliva of the mouth. Bile is produced in the liver and stored in the gallbladder.

20. **(C)** Peristalsis is the coordinated wavelike contraction of the gastrointestinal tract responsible for the movement of food through the system. Pleurisy is inflammation of the parietal pleurae of the lungs. Peritonitis is an inflammatory reaction of the peritoneum. Pyelonephritis is an inflammation of the kidney and renal pelvis caused by bacteria.

21. **(A)** The duodenum is the first part of the small intestine. The next sections are the jejunum and ileum, followed by the cecum of the large bowel.

22. **(C)** A tear of the mesentery may cause a loss of nerve and blood supply to the organ to which it is attached. Bleeding may be severe. Distention can occur from the accumulation of blood. Peritonitis will be caused if stomach contents are allowed into the peritoneal cavity. This can cause severe pain in a patient and may be demonstrated by a "guarded" or rigid abdomen. Peritonitis can lead to death.

23. **(C)** Injuries involving the descending aorta or venae cavae are considered abdominal injuries. Bowel contents released into the peritoneal cavity will cause extreme pain, while blood will have much less effect. Hollow-organ injuries release bowel content and cause severe pain with tenderness and muscle rigidity. Solid organs primarily release blood when injured.

24. **(C)** After you loosen Mr. Kocker's clothing and observe his position (often a clue of underlying causes), you should record his vital signs, as they may be rapidly changing. Early vital signs, especially pulse, blood pressure, and respirations, are indicated in all acute abdomen patients.

25. **(D)** Mr. Kocker will most likely be breathing rapidly and shallowly in order to cause the least painful movement of the abdomen.

26. **(C)** Mr. Kocker's halfmoon-shaped bruise may be from impact with a steering wheel. These bruises often take from 12 to 24 hours after impact to develop. He should be questioned about any recent trauma that might explain his acute abdomen. He may very well be in shock.

27. **(B)** Eviscerations are best cared for by applying sterile dressings moistened with sterile saline, then covering the dressings with sterile aluminum foil and taping them to occlude air from entering. This will prevent drying of the organs and assist in body heat retention.

28. **(D)** A pulsing or throbbing mass palpated during an examination of an acute abdomen is a significant sign, as it may be an aortic aneurysm. Rapid transportation, O_2, and all basic life-support procedures may be required. Peritonitis is rapidly caused by spilled abdominal contents from hollow organs. Foreign objects impaled in the victim should not be removed in the field; stabilize and control bleeding.

29. **(C)** Referred pain arises from the visceral (serosa or mesentery) peritoneum and is conveyed through its autonomic nervous system. The parietal peritoneum (lining of the wall of the abdomen) perceives sensations much like the skin and can localize pain very well. The visceral peritoneum can only sense stretching or distention of the abdomen.

30. **(C)** Peptic ulcers are the most common cause of hematemesis in the United States. Dysphagia is difficulty in swallowing. Esophageal varices are collateral veins in the esophagus that are under extreme pressure and often rupture, producing copious bleeding. Gastritis is an inflammation of the lining of the stomach.

31. **(A)** The loss of body fluid is always associated with peritonitis and can lead to shock. Patients with peritonitis can only vomit to excrete food in the stomach and do so often. High fever is generally not seen in appendicitis until after the appendix has ruptured and infection is introduced into the peritoneal cavity. Abdominal palpation should always be done gently and with warm hands.

32. **(D)** Supplemental O_2 may be administered in cases of acute abdomen as a precaution. If signs of shock are present, all of your technical skills and knowledge may be needed to support the patient. Never give anything by mouth to a patient with a suspected acute abdomen. Never attempt to relieve pain by use of analgesics or narcotics, as it will mask the patient's symptoms in the Emergency Department. Ice packs will do little for the patient.

33. **(B)** Dissected and ruptured aneurysms produce sharp pain in the back and lower right quadrant. The patient will need high-concentration O_2

and legs elevated, and may need CPR. If authorized, the pneumatic counter-pressure device may also be indicated. Appendicitis has referred pain about the navel and direct lower right quadrant pain. Pancreatitis has upper back and abdomen pain. A duodenal ulcer produces direct upper midabdomen or upper back pain.

34. (A) Perforated peptic ulcers produce generalized pain throughout the abdomen. Cholecystitis may show referred right shoulder or direct upper right quadrant pain. Diverticulitis presents lower left quadrant pain. Kidney stones may present on either side, with the pain moving toward the genitalia as the stone moves; this pain is excruciating.

35. (B) A typical source of pain in the lower left quadrant is intestinal obstruction and renal pain. Gastritis, pancreatitis, and myocardial ischemia often present in the upper left quadrant of the abdomen.

36. (B) Hepatitis typically presents pain in the upper right quadrant.

37. (D) A patient with isolated blunt abdominal trauma can be transported in a supine position unless contraindicated by the presence of shock. Assist respiration and use oxygen as needed. Properly worn safety belts can produce injury while absorbing the energy of a deceleration crash. The effect of the belt stretching and dissipating crash forces is called "ride down." A full (distended) bladder is more likely to rupture than an empty one.

38. (C) The ureters connect the kidneys with the urinary bladder. The uterus is a pear-shaped, hollow female reproductive organ. The urethra is the opening to the outside of the body from which urine flows.

39. (B) Renal colic or the "passing of stones" is extremely painful and the patient will be able to tell you exactly where it hurts. The patient's blood pressure will generally remain within normal ranges; the pulse rate will probably be elevated due to the severe pain. There will be profound diaphoresis.

40. (B) A woman of childbearing age presenting an acute abdomen should be questioned regarding her recent history of menstruation. Missed periods may give a clue to a pregnancy, possibly outside of the uterine cavity. This condition could lead to rapid hemorrhaging and shock

should there be a rupture. Pain may be localized to the open side of the abdomen. Transport this patient on her left side, so additional pressure is not placed on the venae cavae, thus reducing venous blood return.

41. (D) Although sexual assault is a serious matter and the victim may be upset, she is still able to give or withdraw consent for treatment. She should be encouraged not to urinate, defecate, or do anything to alter or destroy evidence. EMTs should not examine her genitalia unless she is injured and, if necessary, carefully remove clothing rather than cutting or tearing it off.

42. (A) Direct local pressure will control most bleeding involving the male genitalia. Moist, sterile dressings are indicated to injuries involving either male or female genitalia. Amputated genitalia should be transported in a sterile dressing, placed in a plastic bag, and kept cool. Ice packs may be applied to the perineal area to reduce swelling.

43. (C) Internal female genitalia are seldom injured by pelvic fractures because the genitalia are well protected and small; this would not be true in pregnant women. Kidney damage can occur from rapid deceleration and spinal fractures, as well as from fractured ribs and penetrating injuries. The urinary bladder can be easily torn if distended in a male patient upon impact. Fractures of the pelvis may or may not be present. Never pack anything in the vaginal canal to control bleeding. Direct pressure may be used on surrounding soft-tissue injuries.

10 Medical Emergencies

This chapter focuses on the general topic of medical emergencies. It contains questions relating to heart disease, stroke, chronic obstructive lung disease, diabetes, and epilepsy. The chapter also includes questions regarding your recognition and care of a patient who has ingested, inhaled, or injected poisons. Bites and stings of bees, spiders, snakes, and marine animals are covered, as is food poisoning.

Other questions relate to unconsciousness and its causes, along with a few questions on communicable diseases such as AIDS. This chapter's subject matter will be examined by all certifying bodies, both in written and practical skills examinations.

1. Mr. Kelly, a 72-year-old, is presenting with weakness of the extremities, impaired speech, double vision, and a dry, sore throat. What type of food poisoning should you suspect in Mr. Kelly's case?

   A. Salmonellosis.
   B. Perfringens poisoning.
   C. Staphylococcal poisoning (staph).
   D. Botulism.

2. Select the correct statement regarding smoke inhalation.

   A. Inhaling hot gases is generally less harmful than inhaling cooler smoke.
   B. Treatment of smoke inhalation requires supplemental O_2 and shallow breaths.
   C. Signs of smoke inhalation include regular pulse and deep respirations.
   D. Deep breathing should be recommended to smoke inhalation patients.

3. You are called to the scene of a house fire. Rescue personnel have just removed a male patient. He is unconscious, is moving air, and has major burns on his arms and legs. You should suspect the cause for his unconsciousness is:

   A. Smoke particulate matter.
   B. Burn pain.
   C. Heat inhalation.
   D. Carbon monoxide poisoning.

4. The leading cause of death in the United States is:

   A. Accidents.
   B. Heart disease.
   C. Cancer.
   D. Stroke.

5. A major uncontrollable risk factor of heart disease is:

   A. Hypertension.
   B. Smoking.
   C. Elevated serum cholesterol levels.
   D. Diabetes mellitus.

6. Select the correct statement regarding atherosclerosis.

    A. Atherosclerosis is the thinning of the arterial walls.
    B. Angina pectoris indicates a degree of atherosclerosis.
    C. The arteries of the heart remain the same diameter, whether at rest or under exertion.
    D. Atherosclerosis has little effect on the lumen size of an artery.

7. Select the correct statement regarding angina pectoris.

    A. Angina may be treated with nitroglycerin, as it will relieve pain in 8 to 10 minutes.
    B. Angina is caused by death of the myocardium.
    C. Emotional or physical stress can lead to angina.
    D. Angina generally lasts 10 to 15 minutes.

8. The correct statement about acute myocardial infarction is:

    A. Nearly two-thirds of all patients suffering a myocardial infarction die before they reach the hospital.
    B. Myocardial infarction is more likely to occur in the right ventricle than the left.
    C. The greatest chance of an arrhythmia occurring after an acute myocardial infarction comes at three to five hours after onset.
    D. Death always occurs after an acute MI.

9. From your understanding of congestive heart failure, which of the following statements is true?

    A. CHF is likely to occur the first day after an infarction.
    B. CHF is caused by the heart's inability to pump enough blood.
    C. CHF is seldom associated with pulmonary edema.
    D. CHF will not cause signs of general body swelling (edema).

10. Choose the correct statement regarding the clinical picture of an acute myocardial infarction (AMI).

    A. The pain will be relieved by rest and nitroglycerin.
    B. The pain may last 30 minutes or several hours.
    C. Chest pain is always associated with acute myocardial infarction.
    D. Approximately 25% of patients with AMI develop some type of cardiac dysrhythmia.

11. Pulmonary edema may be caused by an AMI. Which of the following statements is correct?

    A. Pulmonary edema is primarily caused by right ventricle failure.
    B. Transport the pulmonary edema patient in a supine position.
    C. With sudden onset of pulmonary edema, you should suspect an AMI.
    D. Respirations of a patient with pulmonary edema will be slow and deep.

12. General physical findings of a patient with an acute myocardial infarction include:

    A. Rising blood pressure.
    B. Rising pulse rate.
    C. Warm, dry skin.
    D. Slow, deep respirations.

13. Choose the correct statement about patients with prior heart operations or pacemakers.

    A. If a pacemaker dysfunction occurs, the patient will usually exhibit a rapid, regular pulse.
    B. A bypass surgical patient is treated exactly in the same way as other cardiac patients.
    C. Most pacemakers are affected by microwave ovens.
    D. CPR should not be performed on a cardiac arrest patient who has a pacemaker, as it may increase the chance of a lacerated heart.

14. Proper care for a conscious AMI patient would include:

    A. Administering oxygen by nasal cannula only.
    B. Transporting in a supine position.
    C. Recording vitals before and after the use of the siren.
    D. Demonstrating a professional attitude and constant reassurance.

15. Which of the following statements describes signs and symptoms of chronic congestive heart failure?

    A. The patient will experience increased dyspnea when moved from a supine position to a semi-sitting position.
    B. The blood pressure of the patient will be lower than normal.
    C. The heart rate will be slower than normal due to excess fluids.

D. The sound of air bubbling through fluid may be heard in the lungs when using a stethoscope to auscultate the chest.

16. A cerebrovascular accident (CVA) or stroke is:

   A. Most commonly caused by an aneurysm.
   B. Nearly always fatal.
   C. An accident in which there is little hope for recovery.
   D. Generally seen with high blood pressure in the elderly.

17. A stroke caused by the clotting of a cerebral artery will result in a:

   A. Lessening of body function.
   B. Severe headache.
   C. Sudden convulsion.
   D. Rapid loss of consciousness.

18. The most obvious indication that a patient may be experiencing a stroke is:

   A. Hemiplegia.
   B. Difficulty in remembering what he or she had for dinner.
   C. A lowering of blood pressure.
   D. Rapid pulse.

19. Proper care for an unconscious stroke patient should include:

   A. Transporting the patient on the unaffected side if paralysis exists.
   B. Administration of nitroglycerin to promote cerebral vessel dilation.
   C. Calming relatives by explaining the seriousness of the illness at patient's bedside.
   D. Taking a pulse in both carotid arteries and the wrist to check for equality.

20. When assisting a patient in taking nitroglycerin for chest pain, you should encourage the patient to:

   A. Swallow the pill.
   B. Chew the pill.
   C. Place it under the tongue.
   D. Take at least four pills at five-minute intervals.

21. Tenderness in the upper right quadrant without a history of injury would lead you to suspect the presence of a disease or disorder involving the:

    A. Colon.
    B. Stomach.
    C. Gallbladder.
    D. Spleen.

22. A patient with a pulmonary embolism will present with sharp chest pain and:

    A. Slowing pulse.
    B. Rising blood pressure.
    C. Dyspnea which increases with deep inspiration.
    D. Gradual onset.

23. A dissecting aortic aneurysm allows blood to leak between the layers of the vessel, causing a bulge. Select the correct statement regarding aortic aneurysms.

    A. The pain can be relieved by repositioning the patient.
    B. Nitroglycerin will give temporary pain relief for an aneurysm.
    C. Peripheral pulses may be different from each other, or absent.
    D. Onset of pain will be gradual and will come and go.

24. A pulmonary disease in which the air sacs (alveoli) are obstructed by spasm is called:

    A. Asthma.
    B. Edema.
    C. Pneumonia.
    D. Emphysema.

25. Select the correct statement regarding the amount of carbon dioxide in the arterial blood and its effect on breathing for an otherwise normal patient.

    A. If the CO_2 level is below normal, a patient will breathe faster.
    B. If the CO_2 level is higher than normal, a patient will breathe faster.
    C. If the O_2 level is below normal, respirations will increase to blow off gases.

D. If the CO_2 level becomes very low, a patient will become narcotized and breathe very slowly.

26. A barrel-like appearance of the chest should lead you to suspect:

    A. Pulmonary edema.
    B. Asthma.
    C. Emphysema.
    D. Pneumonia.

27. Care for a patient with chronic obstructive lung disease who is experiencing acute dyspnea should include:

    A. Transportation in a recumbent position.
    B. Administration of supplemental O_2 by venturi mask.
    C. Recording vital signs every 15 minutes.
    D. Urging the patient to take shallow breaths.

28. Common signs and symptoms of an acute asthma attack include:

    A. Chest pain.
    B. Lowered pulse rate, lowering blood pressure.
    C. Wheezing on inspiration.
    D. Wheezing on exhalation.

29. A hyperventilating patient without lung abnormalities should be encouraged to breathe into a paper bag. This patient commonly presents with:

    A. High blood pressure.
    B. Numbness or tingling of the hands and feet.
    C. Normal pulse rate.
    D. Chest pains which increase upon exhalation.

30. Causes of hyperventilation include:

    A. Insulin shock.
    B. Ingestion of alkalis.
    C. Pulmonary embolus.
    D. Bronchitis.

31. When treating Reggi, a 37-year-old male, for angina pectoris, you should:

    A. Have him lie down.
    B. Administer low-concentration O_2.
    C. Try to get him to relax.
    D. Give two hypertension medication capsules.

32. Symptoms of diabetes mellitus include:

    A. Hypoxia.
    B. Polydipsia.
    C. Lack of thirst.
    D. Unequal pupils.

33. A patient with signs of diabetic ketoacidosis will have physical signs including:

    A. Full, slow pulse.
    B. High blood pressure.
    C. Normal odor on breath.
    D. Kussmaul's respirations.

34. A patient in insulin shock will present with:

    A. Full, slow pulse.
    B. High blood pressure.
    C. Normal odor on breath.
    D. Kussmaul's respirations.

35. From the following groups of signs and symptoms, select the one that represents those of a person in insulin shock.

    A. Intense thirst, air hunger, diplopia, tremors.
    B. Intense thirst, normal respirations, normal vision, no tremors.
    C. No thirst, air hunger, normal vision, no tremors.
    D. No thirst, normal respirations, diplopia, tremors.

36. Select the correct statement regarding diabetic ketoacidosis.

    A. Administration of sugar will cause rapid improvement.
    B. Exaggerated air hunger will be present as a late symptom.
    C. Ketoacidosis usually has rapid onset.
    D. Pale, moist skin is associated with diabetic ketoacidosis.

37. Some EMS systems use blood glucose reagent strips to test blood sugar levels in the field. Select the most appropriate statement.

    A. You should pin-prick the radial artery for the blood sample.
    B. The blood should be wiped off the reagent strip with an alcohol swab.
    C. Store the reagent strips near a heater outlet in the patient compartment.
    D. Administer some readily available form of glucose if the patient's blood glucose level is below 60 mg/dl.

38. Select the correct statement regarding the general care for a patient suspected of experiencing a diabetic emergency.

    A. Administer sugar to all conscious diabetic emergency patients if you are unsure of their exact condition.
    B. A patient in insulin shock must receive insulin at the Emergency Department to reverse the condition.
    C. "Instant glucose" is highly effective in the treatment of unconscious diabetic patients.
    D. Giving sugar to a patient in diabetic coma will seriously worsen the potential condition.

39. An unconscious patient found with constricted pupils should lead you to suspect:

    A. Alcohol abuse.
    B. Narcotics overdose.
    C. Stroke.
    D. Barbiturate use.

40. A known epileptic patient is observed walking aimlessly, muttering to himself. This type of seizure is classified as:

    A. Simple partial.
    B. Complex partial.
    C. Tonic-clonic.
    D. Generalized.

41. The proper management of a convulsive seizure patient should include:

    A. Placing a padded tongue blade between the front teeth.

B. Placing the patient on his side.
C. Using rigid restraints to protect the extremities.
D. Placing a padded tongue blade between the molars.

42. After a patient experiences a convulsive seizure, you should expect him or her to be:

    A. Oriented.
    B. Postictal.
    C. Breathing rapidly.
    D. Alert and active.

43. General guidelines for the treatment of seizures include:

    A. Transport all known epileptic seizure patients.
    B. Keep seizure patients active after the end of convulsions.
    C. Routinely restrain patients who present aberrant behavior.
    D. Transport patients with recurrent seizures or seizures lasting more than 10 minutes.

44. You are called to an office complex to aid a person who has fainted. Upon your arrival, you find a female who has been unconscious for 20 minutes. You should:

    A. Place a padded tongue blade in her mouth.
    B. Determine if her airway is patent.
    C. Access vital signs before giving any other care.
    D. Immediately administer instant glucose.

45. Your examination of an unconscious patient's clothing reveals a prescription container labeled Reserpine. You should suspect the patient is suffering from:

    A. Diabetes.
    B. Epilepsy.
    C. Alcoholism.
    D. Hypertension.

46. Status epilepticus is defined as a:

    A. Petit mal seizure.
    B. Myoclonic seizure.

C. Patient who has experienced a grand mal seizure.
  D. Series of any type of seizures occurring in rapid succession without periods of consciousness in between.

47. Phenobarbital is commonly used in the treatment of:

    A. Diabetes.
    B. Epilepsy.
    C. Alcoholism.
    D. Hypertension.

48. When called to the scene of a poisoning, your first action should be to:

    A. Give two glasses of water or milk.
    B. Contact the poison control center.
    C. Determine if a poisoning has occurred.
    D. Induce vomiting.

49. Aside from resuscitating a poisoned patient, the most important care you can render is to:

    A. Give syrup of ipecac.
    B. Identify and transport any substance you believe to be the cause of the poisoning.
    C. Give activated charcoal.
    D. Give activated charcoal and syrup of ipecac together.

50. The first rule of emergency care for a patient who has ingested poison is to:

    A. Dilute the poison.
    B. Induce vomiting.
    C. Provide supportive care.
    D. Contact the poison control center.

51. You should induce vomiting if a patient has recently ingested a:

    A. Poison and is convulsing.
    B. Strong acid.
    C. Petroleum product.
    D. Bottle of aspirin.

52. Select the correct statement regarding the induction of vomiting for a patient who has ingested poison.

   A. Administration of syrup of ipecac should be repeated until vomiting occurs.
   B. Syrup of ipecac will normally induce vomiting within 15 to 20 minutes.
   C. To avoid cross-contamination of EMTs, all vomitus should be disposed of appropriately.
   D. The usual dosage of syrup of ipecac is 1 ounce every 20 minutes until vomiting occurs.

53. Select the correct statement regarding the use of activated charcoal with a patient who has ingested poison.

   A. Activated charcoal is used in conjunction with syrup of ipecac.
   B. Activated charcoal is used to absorb the ingested poison in the stomach.
   C. The usual dose of activated charcoal is 4 tablespoons to a large glass of warm water.
   D. Small children's fears may require that activated charcoal be forced into their mouths.

54. Inhaled poisons, such as carbon monoxide and propane, are best treated by the use of:

   A. Compressed air from a self-contained breathing apparatus.
   B. Supplemental O_2.
   C. Syrup of ipecac to stimulate deep breathing.
   D. Activated charcoal to reduce blood gas levels of the toxin.

55. Which statement reflects the correct action for cases involving a contact (surface) poisoning?

   A. Wash off any dry materials.
   B. Attempt to neutralize the material on the skin.
   C. Direct your irrigation stream on the patient's clothes as they are being removed.
   D. Acids can be neutralized on the skin by applying alkalis.

56. You have been dispatched to a one-vehicle rollover on a nearby interstate. The driver of the overturned pickup truck states that he

was transporting phosphorus and you observe a powdery substance on his clothing. Your care for the driver will include:

- A. Immediate irrigation with water.
- B. Covering the man with a burn sheet.
- C. Blowing the powder off his clothing with a dry chemical fire extinguisher.
- D. Removal of all of his clothing making certain not to get the powder wet.

57. Select the correct statement regarding the care of an unconscious patient.

    A. The initial care of an unconscious patient should be to determine the cause.
    B. Any material about the patient, such as plants, drugs, or bottles, should be transported with the patient.
    C. Unconscious patients should be transported in a supine position with legs elevated.
    D. After determining the presence of pulse and respiration, the airway must be opened.

58. Initial care for a patient with a honeybee sting includes:

    A. Removal of the stinger by use of forceps.
    B. Application of hot packs.
    C. Removal of the stinger by scraping it off.
    D. Application of ice packs.

59. Proper management for a patient experiencing a hypersensitive reaction to a bee sting should include first basic life support, then:

    A. Venous tourniquet above the injection site.
    B. Venous tourniquets above and below the injection site.
    C. Warm packs over the injection site.
    D. Ice packs over injection site.

60. Select the proper statement regarding spider bites.

    A. A brown recluse spider bite produces systemic manifestations and often causes death.
    B. A black widow spider bite causes severe local tissue damage.

C. Venom from a black widow spider bite causes tightness in the chest, sweating, and severe muscle cramps.
D. There is no antivenin available for black widow spider bites.

61. A dog bite is a common injury in the United States. Most people are very concerned with the potential of developing rabies. It can be said that:

    A. Rabies can be carried only by dogs.
    B. Any dog that bites a person must be killed and taken to the health department.
    C. Antibiotics prevent the development of rabies.
    D. A rabid dog may act perfectly normal.

62. Emergency care for a patient bitten by a pit viper includes:

    A. Immediate incision of the skin over the fang marks.
    B. Determining if envenomization has occurred.
    C. Rapid transportation, as death is likely.
    D. Application of ice packs and elevation if a limb is bitten.

63. Choose the correct statement regarding a coral snake bite.

    A. A coral snake bite exhibits many local manifestations, including massive swelling and a large area of discoloration.
    B. A coral snake bite should be incised and the venom sucked out.
    C. A coral snake bite is toxic to the brain, causing paralysis of respiration and eyes.
    D. A coral snake-bitten extremity should be packed in ice.

64. General care for a patient suffering a sting from a marine animal includes:

    A. Applying ice.
    B. Covering the affected area with a sterile dressing.
    C. Sprinkling the affected area with alcohol, meat tenderizer, and talcum powder.
    D. Incising and sucking out venom around the affected area.

65. Punctures from the spines of catfish, urchins, and sting rays should be cared for by:

    A. Applying ice.

B. Sprinkling the affected area with alcohol, meat tenderizer, and talcum powder.
C. Incising the area around the puncture and sucking out the venom.
D. Immobilizing the affected area and soaking in hot water.

66. Carbon monoxide poisoning can have many causes, including exhaust fumes from cars, sewer gases, and charcoal grills. Select the correct statement regarding CO poisonings.

    A. A headache, slight dizziness, or weakness may be present.
    B. CO poisonings take at least one hour of exposure to be fatal.
    C. Treatment requires little more than removal of the patient from the poisonous environment.
    D. CO smells and tastes like rotten eggs.

67. The general care for a conscious patient who has ingested a poisonous plant would be to:

    A. Dilute the poison.
    B. Immobilize the ingested plant by the use of activated charcoal.
    C. Induce vomiting.
    D. Use a specific antidote for each type of plant ingested.

68. A common sign or symptom of iron tablet poisoning is:

    A. Respiratory distress.
    B. Elevated blood pressure.
    C. Warm skin.
    D. Bright red blood in diarrhea or emesis.

69. Characteristic symptoms of ingested drain cleaner include:

    A. Burns about the lips and mouth.
    B. Deep respirations.
    C. Hot skin temperature.
    D. Prompt vomiting of the substance by the patient.

70. A patient suspected of ingesting a large quantity of salicylates (aspirin) will present with:

    A. Lack of thirst.
    B. Rapid, deep breathing.
    C. Lowered body temperature.
    D. Dry skin.

71. Immediate onset of paralysis will result from:

    A. Gradual compression of the spinal cord.
    B. A completely severed spinal cord.
    C. Ingested poison.
    D. A coral snake bite.

72. Ingestion of arsenic would cause a/an:

    A. Garlic breath odor.
    B. Hot, dry skin.
    C. Lack of thirst.
    D. Intense hunger.

73. Select the correct statement about the ingestion of "D-Con" rat poison.

    A. Symptoms will occur after 1 hour.
    B. Vomiting should not be induced with this type of poisoning.
    C. Vomiting will occur spontaneously after ingestion.
    D. Back and abdominal pain and blood in the urine and stool may present 24 to 36 hours after ingestion.

74. On a hot summer afternoon, you are called for an unknown illness. You discover a 46-year-old female unconscious on the floor of her office. Your exam reveals a medic alert tag stating allergies to bee stings. A co-worker tells you she has been drinking heavily and using drugs. She has wheezing respirations, hives, a blood pressure of 94/50, and a strong odor of alcohol. You should suspect:

    A. Amphetamine overdose.
    B. Anaphylactic shock.
    C. Alcohol overdose.
    D. Marijuana overdose.

75. Many terms are used when discussing communicable diseases. Select the correct statement below.

    A. Contamination refers to the disease state in a person.
    B. A carrier is an infected person.
    C. A host is a source of infection.
    D. A reservoir cannot be a source of infection.

76. Proper infection control procedures for a known AIDS patient include the use of:

    A. Disposable gloves.
    B. Occlusive dressing on all AIDS victims' wounds.
    C. Stainless steel suction catheter.
    D. Soapy hot water mixture for blood cleanup.

77. When caring for a patient with AIDS, you should also:

    A. Have the patient wear a mask.
    B. Destroy linens after use.
    C. Remove the ambulance from service for 24 hours after transporting an AIDS patient.
    D. Discard nondisposable items.

78. Select the correct statement regarding hepatitis.

    A. Viral hepatitis should be suspected in patients with "needle tracks" on their arms.
    B. Serum hepatitis is transmitted in fecal contaminants.
    C. Gamma globulin shots may be recommended if the EMT is exposed to viral hepatitis.
    D. Handwashing will do little to prevent the EMT from contracting viral hepatitis.

79. After transporting a patient with a known communicable disease, you should:

    A. Air the ambulance for 30 minutes.
    B. Scrub the ambulance with soap and water.
    C. Scrub the ambulance and towel dry all exposed surfaces.
    D. Disinfect exposed surfaces and allow them to air dry.

80. The EMT is exposed to communicable disease on a frequent basis. The best precaution an EMT can take to avoid infection is to:

    A. Use disposable equipment.
    B. Scrub the ambulance once a day.
    C. Wear a mask and gown.
    D. Have regular exams and up-to-date immunization.

Answers with Rationale

1. **(D)** Mr. Kelly's symptoms of double vision, impaired speech, weakness, and a dry, sore throat can have many causes. Botulism should be suspected if no other history, such as stroke, is present. Most other types of food poisoning are associated with diarrhea, nausea, abdominal cramps, and, often, vomiting.

2. **(B)** Treatment of smoke inhalation requires supplemental O_2 and, if the patient can cooperate, shallow breaths. Shallow breathing reduces the number of particles reaching the lower airways. Deep exhalation may also expel some particulate matter. Inhalation of hot gas causes severe swelling and may occlude the upper airway. Smoke inhalation patients experience shortness of breath, wheezing, and a rapid or irregular pulse.

3. **(D)** The unconsciousness of the patient just rescued from a house fire is most likely caused by carbon monoxide poisoning. The patient should receive high-concentration O_2. Superheated air would probably occlude the upper airways. Major burns alone are generally not painful enough to cause a loss of consciousness. Smoke particulate matter will clog the lower airways and can lead to unconsciousness, but CO is the most likely cause.

4. **(B)** While accidents are the leading cause of death for age group 1–44, diseases of the heart are the leading cause of death in the United States, followed by cancer and strokes.

5. **(D)** An uncontrollable risk factor of heart disease is diabetes. Hypertension, serum cholesterol levels, and smoking can be corrected by medication or changing a patient's habits.

6. **(B)** Angina pectoris indicates the presence of atherosclerosis. It reduces the lumen size (inside diameter) of the coronary vessels by thickening of the vessel walls through the accumulation of calcium and fatty deposits. The coronary arteries dilate during exertion.

7. **(C)** Emotional or physical stress can cause angina. Angina usually lasts 3 to 8 minutes and is rapidly relieved by the use of nitroglycerin, usu-

ally within 1 to 2 minutes after administration. Angina is not a sign of death in the myocardium but rather a sign of reduced oxygenation. Pain lasting more than 10 minutes indicates a possible myocardial infarction.

8. (A) Nearly two-thirds of all patients suffering an acute MI die before they reach the hospital. The infarction is more likely to occur in the left side of the heart. The greatest possibility of arrhythmias occurring is in the first hour after an MI. Basic life support can do much to prevent sudden death of acute MI patients in cardiac arrest especially if early defibrillation is provided in the field.

9. (B) Congestive heart failure is caused by the heart's inability to pump enough blood. Left ventricle failure causes a decrease of blood return from the lungs, creating an excess of fluid in the lung alveoli or pulmonary edema. Pulmonary edema may rapidly become present in a patient with left ventricle failure. General body swelling will also occur as venous blood circulation is reduced.

10. (B) The pain associated with an acute MI may last 30 minutes to several hours. It will not be relieved by nitroglycerin. Nearly 90% of all acute MI patients develop some sort of cardiac dysrhythmia. Chest pain does not always mean death of the myocardium. It can indicate angina or a pulmonary problem such as a pulmonary embolus.

11. (C) Sudden onset of pulmonary edema without history of trauma should always lead you to suspect an acute MI. It is generally caused by left ventricle failure. The patient will breathe shallowly and rapidly and should be transported with the head elevated. This will reduce the venous blood return that is aggravating the condition. Administer O_2 liberally.

12. (B) Generally, an acute MI patient will present with a rising pulse rate, as the heart tries to compensate for the tissue hypoxia. The blood pressure may fall; the skin will be cool and moist. Respirations will be normal unless pulmonary edema is present, in which case they will be rapid and shallow.

13. (B) Regardless of the presence of pacemakers or bypass surgery, all cardiac patients must be cared for in the same manner. If cardiac arrest is present, CPR must be instituted to preserve life. Failing pacemakers usually exhibit a rapid or irregular pulse. Modern pacemakers are not

affected by microwave ovens. CPR presents no danger of further injury to a heart in which a pacemaker has been placed.

14. (D) A professional attitude and constant reassurance will do much to reduce the fears of an acute MI patient. Panic constricts blood vessels; any action that reduces panic is therapeutic. O_2 should be administered by mask to achieve higher concentrations. The patient should be transported in a semi-sitting position to aid in comfort. The vitals should be recorded frequently, but the siren should probably not be used because it will add to the patient's anxiety, thus increasing the workload of an already overtaxed heart.

15. (D) Patients with congestive heart failure tend to have wet lungs, easily heard by auscultation of the chest. The heart rate will increase to reduce the congestion in the lungs. Blood pressure will be normal or slightly elevated. The patient will be most comfortable in a sitting position, as lying down returns venous blood to the heart and lungs, aggravating the congestion.

16. (D) Generally speaking, high blood pressure is seen in elderly stroke patients. The most common cause of a stroke is clotting of a cerebral arterial vessel. Strokes are seldom fatal, and there is great hope for partial or complete recovery.

17. (A) A stroke caused by the clotting of a cerebral artery will result in a lessening of body function. Severe headache, sudden convulsion, or rapid loss of consciousness may indicate a stroke caused by an arterial rupture. Protect the patient experiencing a convulsion by clearing the area around him of any objects he might accidentally strike.

18. (A) A stroke patient often exhibits hemiplegia (paralysis on one side of the body). The blood pressure will probably be high, the pulse slow.

19. (D) Take a pulse in both carotid arteries and at the wrist to check for presence and equality of pressure. Do not check both carotids at the same time. Nitroglycerin is used for angina. It will do little for a stroke patient. The patients should have supplemental O_2 administered. Transport on the affected side, remembering to protect the patient while moving. Try to avoid discussing an unconscious patient's condition around him or her. A seemingly unconscious patient is often aware of

surroundings. Try to keep relatives calm to reduce possible patient anxiety.

20. (C) Nitroglycerin should be placed under the tongue, where it will be rapidly absorbed. Nitroglycerin is generally not given more than three times at three- to five-minute intervals. If no effect is seen, either the medication has deteriorated or the condition is more extensive than angina.

21. (C) Gallbladder disease is often signaled by tenderness in the upper right quadrant and can be present without trauma.

22. (C) A patient with a pulmonary embolism will present with dyspnea and sharp pain which increases with deep inspiration. The onset will be sudden, the pulse rate will rise, and the blood pressure may fall. Acute cor pulmonale has very similar symptoms and is treated in the same manner.

23. (C) Peripheral pulses may be different or even absent in a patient with a dissecting aortic aneurysm. Pain will be sudden in onset and persistent. Body positioning or nitroglycerin will not relieve the pain.

24. (A) In the disease process of asthma, the air sacs are obstructed by spasms of the large airways. Air sacs are damaged by the presence of edema (fluid), pneumonia (infection), or emphysema (mucus).

25. (B) If the CO_2 level in the blood is higher than normal, an otherwise normal patient will breathe faster to "blow off" the excess. Should the CO_2 level fall below normal, a patient will breathe slower to replenish it. If the CO_2 level becomes extremely high, the respiratory center becomes narcotized or depressed. The secondary respiratory drive will be activated. This is a response to a low O_2 level in the blood.

26. (C) Patients with emphysema (chronic obstructive lung disease) generally develop a barrel-like appearance of the chest. This is very common in emphysema patients, who tend to be thin, and usually smoke.

27. (B) Supplemental O_2 should be administered to COLD patients by venturi mask. Oxygen use should be closely monitored, as its use may reduce the patient's respiratory drive. If cyanosis is present, increase O_2 level and be prepared to assist the patient by using positive-pressure

ventilation. The patient will probably be most comfortable in a sitting or nearly upright position. Respiratory rate should be checked at least every five minutes to monitor proper O_2 delivery levels.

28. (D) Commonly, asthma patients wheeze on exhalation. Their problem is not getting air in, but getting air out. Chest pain is seldom present in asthma. The pulse rate will be normal; the blood pressure may be elevated.

29. (B) Hyperventilation syndrome will cause numbness or tingling in the hands or feet as excessive amounts of CO_2 are blown off. The blood pressure will remain normal and the pulse rate will increase. Stabbing chest pains may be present and will increase during inspiration.

30. (C) Causes of hyperventilation include pulmonary embolus and ingestion of acids. The respirations increase as the body tries to blow off the acid in the blood. Diabetic coma (ketoacidosis) can also cause hyperventilation as the body attempts to rid itself of excess acid.

31. (C) A patient suffering an angina pectoris attack should be encouraged to remain as calm as possible. The patient will probably be most comfortable sitting up. High-concentration O_2 may be of benefit.

32. (B) Both polydipsia (frequent drinking of liquids) and polyuria (frequent urination) are symptoms of diabetes. Thirst and the frequent drinking of liquids are caused by the need to replenish fluids as the urine is used to wash away excess amounts of sugar. These patients do not have unequal pupils.

33. (D) Kussmaul's respirations (rapid, deep sighing) are characteristic of ketoacidosis. The pulse will be rapid and weak. The blood pressure may be normal or low. The odor of the breath may resemble acetone (sweet, fruity).

34. (C) The odor of the breath is usually normal. Insulin shock will present with normal respirations, normal blood pressure, and a full, rapid pulse.

35. (D) A patient in early stages of insulin shock (hypoglycemia) will exhibit no thirst (probably drooling), have normal respirations and

diplopia (double vision), and possibly be in tremors. The more advanced patient may be irritable, in seizures, or in a coma.

36. (B) A later sign of ketoacidosis is exaggerated air hunger, which occurs as the body tries to blow off CO_2. Administration of sugar will do nothing to improve the patient's condition, nor will it worsen it. Ketoacidosis will be gradual in onset, often taking several days. The skin will be warm and dry.

37. (D) A low blood glucose level (below 60 mg/dl) should be aggressively corrected. A urine test for ketone is also indicated. The reagent strips are susceptible to deterioration from moisture, heat, and light. Check with a pharmacist for restocking guidelines. Capillary blood from a prick of the palmar surface of the patient's finger is used for *Chemstrip bG* testing.

38. (A) Administration of sugar is indicated in all diabetic emergency patients when you are unsure of their exact condition. Sugar may save the life of a patient in insulin shock. It will do little harm to a person in diabetic coma. Instant glucose-type preparations are not as effectively absorbed by the mouth as previously believed. Sugar cubes may endanger the airway and should be used with great caution.

39. (B) Narcotic overdose often causes constriction of the pupils. Use of alcohol and barbiturates causes dilated or sluggish pupils. A stroke may cause a pupil to dilate.

40. (B) A patient observed walking aimlessly, muttering to himself, may be experiencing a complex partial seizure. A simple partial seizure may be limited to one or two extremities or one side of the body. A tonic-clonic or generalized seizure involves the entire body.

41. (B) The proper management of a convulsive seizure patient should include positioning the patient on the side, and only restraining the patient to prevent serious self-injury. Never place a bite stick or your finger between the front teeth, because the stick may break the teeth or your finger may be cut.

42. (B) The patient will generally be lethargic, sleepy, and breathing slowly after the end of a convulsive seizure (postictal). Let the patient rest and return to normal respiratory levels at this point.

43. (D) Patients with recurrent seizures or seizures lasting more than 10 minutes should be transported for thorough examination at the Emergency Department. Known seizure patients may not require transportation if they are uninjured and resting after a short seizure.

44. (B) Airway maintenance is your first priority. The female patient in this question has been unconscious for some period of time. Simple fainting (syncope) is probably not the condition that exists, as she should have experienced a rapid return to consciousness. If a medic alert card or tag is noted, with diabetes listed as a condition, sugar may be administered orally only if the patient is conscious enough to swallow. Vital signs may give a clue as to her malady and are indicated early on in the treatment of unconscious patients.

45. (D) Reserpine is a drug used for the control of hypertension. Other common drugs are Orinase and Diabinese, used by diabetics.

46. (D) Status epilepticus is defined as a series of seizures occurring in rapid succession in which the patient does not regain consciousness between seizures. This is a very dangerous condition, as the brain may not be adequately perfused, aggravating the seizure problem. This condition could lead to death.

47. (B) Phenobarbital, Dilantin, and Mysoline are used in the treatment of epilepsy.

48. (C) Your first action at the scene of a poisoning call should be to determine if a poisoning has actually occurred. Often a parent only suspects that a child has ingested a toxin. Careful questioning of frantic parents may lead to the discovery that a poisoning has not actually taken place.

49. (B) Aside from providing supportive care, such as airway maintenance or CPR, you can do much to save a life by determining the type and amount of poison to which a patient has been exposed. Transport suspect materials to the Emergency Department for accurate identification.

50. (C) The first rule of emergency care for a person who has ingested poison is to provide any supportive care indicated. Protection of the airway, adequate ventilation, and CPR may be indicated. After this priority has been addressed, contact either the poison control center or your

Medical Control for further instructions before diluting the poison with one or two glasses of milk or water.

51. (D) Generally speaking, vomiting should be induced as soon as possible in a conscious patient who has ingested large quantities of aspirin. Aspirin can take several hours to be absorbed by the digestive system. Vomiting should not be induced in cases where a corrosive (acid or alkali) or petroleum product (lighter fluid, gasoline, kerosene) has been ingested. A high danger of additional burns and aspiration exists. A patient unable to protect the airway, such as a semiconscious or unconscious person, should not have vomiting induced. Local protocols should always be followed with regard to the inducement of vomiting.

52. (B) Syrup of ipecac will normally induce vomiting in 15 to 20 minutes. Ipecac should be followed by a glass of clear liquid (warm water may be beneficial). The dose will vary with the weight of the patient. If vomiting does not occur, one additional dose may be given. Collect all vomitus (emesis) in a plastic bag and deliver to the Emergency Department staff for evaluation. Generally, the EMT should not induce vomiting until directed to do so by either the poison control center or Medical Control.

53. (B) Activated charcoal is used to absorb ingested poisons in the stomach. Activated charcoal should not be given with syrup of ipecac, as it will absorb the ipecac and halt its effect. The usual dose of activated charcoal is 1 tablespoon thoroughly mixed in a glass of water. Activated charcoal should not be forced into a patient's mouth, as this may cause airway problems or promote vomiting.

54. (B) Removal from the contaminated area and high-concentration O_2 is indicated in cases of inhaled noxious gases. Syrup of ipecac and activated charcoal are used for ingested poisons only.

55. (C) For a patient exposed to a contact poison, prompt removal of the offending substance is indicated. Direct your irrigation stream on the patient's clothing as it is removed, not at the skin since high pressure could tear tissue. Dust off any dry material before irrigating, as water may activate the substance or cause burns to the patient. Do not attempt to neutralize contact poisons; irrigate with copious amounts of water.

56. (D) Phosphorus, sodium, and potassium are examples of water-reactive flammable solids. Spontaneous ignition is likely when these elements become moist or wet with water. Other chemicals can produce flammable gases if they come in contact with water. Extreme caution including observation of hazardous materials placards from a distance is always appropriate when a chance of hazard exists.

57. (B) Any material found in the area of an unconscious patient should be transported to the Emergency Department for identification. Oftentimes, the physician can identify a possible cause for the patient's condition from this evidence. The initial care for an unconscious patient is always to establish the airway first, with later attention to the possible cause of unconsciousness. Unconscious patients should be transported in a coma position unless contraindicated by spinal injury or some other condition.

58. (C) Initial care for honeybee stings includes removing the implanted stinger by scraping it off with a knife or fingernail. Do not use forceps, as this may cause additional venom to be injected into the skin. Applying ice after the stinger has been removed may reduce the pain and swelling.

59. (B) Venous tourniquets applied above and below the site of a honeybee sting may reduce the absorption of venom. A hypersensitive patient may experience breathing difficulties and other signs of anaphylactic shock, including cardiac arrest. After the venous tourniquets, you then apply ice packs over the injection site to reduce the rate at which venom is absorbed. Local policies will determine if you can administer epinephrine to such a patient. A subcutaneous injection of 0.3–0.5 mL of 1:1000 epinephrine may be ordered.

60. (C) Black widow spider venom causes severe muscle cramps, sweating, and tightness of the chest. There is a specific antivenin available for black widow spider bites. Local tissue damage will be minimal from a black widow spider bite, but rather severe from a bite of a brown recluse spider. Deaths caused by the bite of a brown recluse spider are rare even though it is a common inhabitant of the United States.

61. (D) A rabid dog may act perfectly normal, or may exhibit signs of abnormal behavior and salivate. Rabies can also be carried by skunks, squirrels, bats, foxes, and raccoons. Do not kill a suspect dog, but en-

courage that it be kept alive and taken to the health department for observation and examination. Antibiotics will not prevent rabies.

62. (B) Emergency care for a patient bitten by a pit viper (rattlesnake, cottonmouth, or copperhead) includes determining if envenomization has actually taken place. Envenomization occurs in about 70% of such cases. Envenomization will cause a burning pain at the injection site within 5 to 10 minutes. Swelling and discoloration will also begin within this time period. Incision of the skin is not indicated unless transport time will take many hours after the envenomization. If an extremity has been involved, immobilize, keep at level of heart or below and apply light constriction bands above and below the wound. Apply cool packs only under medical direction.

63. (C) A coral snake bite is toxic to the brain and causes paralysis of respiration, eyes, and eyelids. Few local manifestations will be noted from a coral snake bite. The skin should not be incised to remove venom. Do not pack an extremity in ice. *Remember*: Red stripes bordering yellow stripes indicate a coral snake.

64. (C) Generally, marine animal stings can be treated by sprinkling the affected area with alcohol (fixes the stinger), meat tenderizer (neutralizes toxin), and talcum powder (dries cells for easy removal). Do not use fresh water on marine animal stings, as it increases the pain. Ice packs may help reduce swelling, but don't get the affected area wet. Incision is not indicated.

65. (D) Puncture wounds from the spines of sea urchins, sting rays, and catfish should be soaked in hot water for 30 to 60 minutes. Immobilize or keep the affected area still. The toxins of these fish are heat-sensitive and pain may abate rapidly.

66. (A) A patient with carbon monoxide poisoning may experience a headache, slight dizziness, or general weakness after a short period of exposure. CO poisoning is rapid and can cause death within minutes. High concentration of humidified O_2 is required for treatment of CO poisoning. CO is odorless and tasteless.

67. (C) Generally, patients who have ingested poisonous plants are treated by inducing vomiting. Your poison control center will give you specific

instructions depending on the material ingested. Transportation should not be delayed for vomiting. Have suction available in case it is needed.

68. (D) A common sign of iron tablet poisoning is bright red blood in diarrhea or vomitus. This may occur within two hours of ingestion. Upper abdominal pain may be severe. Signs of shock may follow significant blood loss.

69. (A) Characteristic signs of ingestion of a strong corrosive, such as drain cleaner, include burns about the lips and mouth. Careful examination of these tissues can confirm ingestion. Respirations will be shallow and the skin may be cold and clammy. Do not induce vomiting in a patient who has ingested a strong corrosive. Contact the poison control center or your Medical Control for further instructions.

70. (B) A patient who has ingested a large quantity of salicylates (aspirin) will present with rapid, deep breathing, extreme thirst, an elevated body temperature, and sweating.

71. (B) A completely severed spinal cord will produce instant paralysis of organs or muscles associated with the cord below the lesion. Gradual compression of the cord, poisonings, and coral snake bites may cause a gradual onset of paralysis.

72. (A) Ingestion of excessive amounts of arsenic will cause garlic-odored breath. The skin will be cold and clammy. There will be vomiting and intense thirst. Burning pains in the stomach and esophagus are also common.

73. (D) Ingestion of "D-Con" rat poison may cause back and abdominal pain and blood in the urine and stool. These symptoms usually take 24–36 hours after ingestion to appear. Vomiting should be induced if it is within an hour after ingestion. Vomiting would be of no value after the poison has been in the body for several hours.

74. (B) The woman has probably been stung by a bee. She is demonstrating signs of anaphylactic shock (wheezing respirations, hives, low blood pressure). Her condition is complicated by her drug use, which will depress her respirations.

75. (C) A host is an infected person or animal that is a source of infection to others. Infection is the term used to describe a state of disease. A carrier is not infected but does transmit the disease. A reservoir is a place where infectious organisms live.

76. (A) Health care workers who come in contact with known AIDS victims should wear disposable gowns and gloves. Thorough handwashing is a must. Sodium hypochlorite (1:10 dilution of household bleach with cool water) is recommended for cleanup of blood, fecal material, and other secretions. Do not put pencils, pens, or other objects in your mouth (this is good general infection control advice). Use disposable equipment whenever possible and dispose of with special warning "Blood Precautions." Even dry, chapped hands can have open areas through which disease-causing organisms such as hepatitis can enter.

77. (A) Since the AIDS patient has an impaired immune system, it may be advisable for the patient to wear a mask to protect himself or herself from the microorganisms present on health care workers and in the ambulance. Linens should be placed in a designated laundry bag for proper laundering. The ambulance should be aired and contact areas should be scrubbed and disinfected with a fresh mixture of 1:10 solution of household bleach and water. Wear gloves while cleaning the ambulance and any time you may contact the patient's bodily fluids.

78. (C) Gamma globulin shots may be recommended to prevent viral hepatitis. Viral hepatitis is passed through the handling of fecal-soiled linens and clothing. Washing the hands can do much to prevent oral contamination. Many communicable diseases are introduced through the mouth. (When was the last time you had a snack after delivering a patient to the Emergency Department?) Serum hepatitis is present in the host's blood. Potential for contamination can exist if you have open lesions (bruises, cuts, etc.) and apply dressings to trauma patients with hepatitis. Serum hepatitis can be suspected in patients with "needle tracks."

79. (D) After transporting a patient with a known communicable disease, the ambulance should be scrubbed with bleach solution and allowed to air dry.

80. (D) The best precaution an EMT can take to avoid personal infection is having regular exams and up-to-date immunization. Use of disposable equipment will reduce the chance of infection to EMTs and future patients. A mask and gown will reduce the chance of infection from known hosts. The ambulance should be thoroughly scrubbed and disinfected at least once a week.

11 Pediatric Emergencies and Childbirth

This chapter's questions on pediatrics are presented to help you recognize and treat many injuries and illnesses common to young people. It is important to keep in mind that children are not just small adults. Pediatric emergencies require specific and unique reactions on the part of the EMT.

This chapter also provides a strong basis for evaluating your skills that pertain to common complications of childbirth and assisting with an uncomplicated, unscheduled childbirth. The APGAR scoring system is also reviewed in this section.

1. Infants, children, and adults are classified by their chronological ages. Select the correct statement defining age categories.

    A. Adults are generally age 14 or older.
    B. Infants are generally less than 1 year old.
    C. Children are 2 years to 12 years old.
    D. Infants are up to 2½ years old.

2. Which of the following generally affects only children under age 3?

    A. Asthma.
    B. Croup.
    C. Epiglottitis.
    D. Emphysema.

3. You are called to the home of a 4-year-old child. The patient has a high fever, and is experiencing pain swallowing. He is sitting, leaning forward, and drooling. You suspect he is suffering from:

    A. Asthma.
    B. Croup.
    C. Epiglottitis.
    D. Emphysema.

4. Care for a child with an airway obstruction suspected of being croup or epiglottitis should include:

    A. Four back blows and four chest thrusts.
    B. Examination of the airway by finger and use of a tongue blade.
    C. Placing the patient in a shock position and transporting.
    D. Administration of high levels of O_2 in a sitting position.

5. The best artery to monitor the pulse rate of a neonate is the:

    A. Carotid.
    B. Brachial.
    C. Radial.
    D. Femoral.

6. A 3-year-old girl is found having a seizure; the skin is hot and flushing. You should:

    A. Give an ice-water bath.
    B. Give a tepid-water sponge bath.

C. Cool the child until she begins to shiver.
D. Take an oral temperature.

7. When examining a child who has been involved in a motor vehicle accident, it is probably most important to:

   A. Avoid inflicting any pain while examining for injuries.
   B. Use simple language to communicate with the child.
   C. Separate the parents from the child to bring calm to the situation.
   D. Cover all open wounds as rapidly as possible.

8. Behavioral indicators of a child that you suspect has been abused include:

   A. Desire to return home.
   B. Wariness of adults.
   C. No reaction to other children's crying.
   D. Desire to stay at home rather than go to school.

9. When caring for a child you suspect has been abused, you should:

   A. Transport to the Emergency Department even if the parents don't want you to do so.
   B. Challenge the parents' actions to determine if the child has been abused.
   C. Report your suspicions to the Emergency Department physician.
   D. Ask the parents to describe the conditions under which the different injuries occurred if they are in many different stages of healing.

10. The average vital signs for a 6-year-old child are:

    A. Pulse 100–140; BP 96/66; resp 30–40.
    B. Pulse 90–110; BP 98/64; resp 20–30.
    C. Pulse 80–100; BP 100/56; resp 20–25.
    D. Pulse 70–110; BP 112/58; resp 14–26.

11. When taking a blood pressure in a child, a blood pressure cuff:

    A. Will produce a high reading if it is too wide.
    B. Should cover about two-thirds of the upper arm.
    C. Will produce a low reading if it is too narrow.
    D. Should be applied only to the thigh.

12. Sudden Infant Death Syndrome (SIDS) accounts for nearly 10,000 deaths per year in the United States. Select the correct statement regarding SIDS.

    A. SIDS babies do not suffocate on blankets or pillows.
    B. SIDS is contagious, and other children should never be exposed to potential SIDS patients.
    C. SIDS is hereditary.
    D. CPR will generally revive a potential SIDS patient.

13. Two-year-old Charlie has eaten half a bottle of his grandmother's ferrous sulfate tablets. You are 30 miles from the hospital. You should:

    A. Transport immediately.
    B. Give Charlie syrup of ipecac.
    C. Give Charlie activated charcoal.
    D. Do nothing because vitamins are nonpoisonous.

14. The third stage of labor:

    A. Begins when contractions are 5 minutes apart.
    B. Begins with the birth of the baby and ends with the delivery of the placenta.
    C. Ends with the delivery of the placenta.
    D. Begins when the cervix is fully dilated and ends when the baby is born.

15. Guidelines for transporting a woman in labor from her home include:

    A. Transporting during the delivery of the placenta if longer than 5 minutes after the birth of the child.
    B. Not transporting if contractions are less than 10 minutes apart.
    C. Remaining at her home if contractions are 2 or 3 minutes apart.
    D. Remaining at her home until the third stage of delivery is completed, regardless of time, unless baby appears distressed.

16. An emergency predelivery condition involving a pregnant patient with hemorrhaging from the vagina caused by an abnormal location of the placenta is called:

    A. Abruptio placentae.
    B. Eclampsia.

C. Primigravida.
D. Placenta previa.

17. A pregnant woman experiencing convulsions during the later stages of pregnancy should:

    A. Be placed on her left side with her head elevated and transported.
    B. Have her blood pressure monitored very closely, as convulsions at such a stage generally indicate hypotension.
    C. Have her vagina examined for any signs of a "bloody show."
    D. Have her abdomen palpated to determine if the fetus is also convulsing, as this may indicate a birth defect of the fetus that is causing the mother's convulsions.

18. The first action you would perform for a pregnant patient not in labor but bleeding heavily from her vagina would be:

    A. Packing the vagina with 2 or 3 sanitary pads.
    B. Transporting the woman on her side with her head elevated 30 to 40 degrees.
    C. Administering high-concentration O_2.
    D. Administering low-concentration O_2, as the fetus may experience oxygen toxicity after five minutes of high-concentration O_2 delivery.

19. Upon arriving at the scene of an emergency childbirth call, you must determine if delivery is imminent. Several questions can be asked of the mother to help you decide whether or not to deliver at the scene. You ask her how she feels. Select the response which would best indicate imminent delivery.

    A. "This is my first baby. I'm O.K."
    B. "I think I am about to have the baby."
    C. "My back really hurts and contractions are three minutes apart."
    D. "I don't feel that I need to go to the bathroom right now."

20. During an emergency delivery outside the hospital setting, you are responsible for positioning a pregnant patient to aid her in the delivery and make her comfortable. Select the statement that describes proper positioning.

    A. The patient should be on a firm surface, with legs apart and head down 8 to 10 inches to prevent shock.

B. There should be about 2 feet of surface area beyond the patient's buttocks on which to place the baby.
C. The patient's feet should be positioned together and knees pulled apart for proper rotation of the hips.
D. The patient should be on a bed with four pillows under her head and two pillows under her buttocks.

21. When the head of the baby begins to push out of the vagina during a contraction, you should:

    A. Encourage the woman to breathe deeply and slowly.
    B. Gently pull the vagina open from both sides to allow passage of the baby.
    C. Apply gentle pressure to the baby's head, using the palm of your hand.
    D. Slide your finger past the baby's head and check for the possibility of the umbilical cord around the baby's neck.

22. You should suction the airway of a newborn baby:

    A. After the entire body is delivered.
    B. Applied to the mouth first.
    C. Applied to the nose first.
    D. As soon as the nose is visible, as babies are primarily nose breathers.

23. After a baby has been born, you should immediately:

    A. Place the baby on the table and re-suction.
    B. Place the baby on the mother's abdomen.
    C. Cut the umbilical cord.
    D. Pick the baby up by the ankles and hang upside down to allow drainage of excess fluids from its airways.

24. Care for the umbilical cord generally begins after a baby is born, has an adequate airway, and is breathing on his or her own. An exception would be if the cord were found around the infant's neck. Choose the correct statement regarding umbilical cord care following a normal delivery.

    A. The cord should be double-clamped, then cut and tied.

B. The cord should be tied, clamped on each side of the tie, and then cut.
   C. The cord should be clamped, tied on each side of the clamp, and then cut.
   D. The cord should be clamped, tied, cut on the mother's side of the tie, and clamped.

25. After the delivery of the infant and the cutting of the cord, your attention can be directed to the delivery of the placenta. Your actions should include:
   A. Transportation at this point, as the baby is out of danger.
   B. Observation of blood loss, which is generally safe if the amount does not exceed 2 pints.
   C. Massaging the uterus until it becomes firm once the placenta delivers.
   D. Packing of the vagina with sanitary napkins if bleeding exceeds one-half pint.

26. After the delivery of the placenta, you should:
   A. Note the exact time of its birth.
   B. Lower the mother's legs and hang them dependent off the table or litter.
   C. Collect all parts of the placenta and deliver them to the Emergency Department along with the infant and mother.
   D. Administer low-concentration O_2 to the mother if bleeding persists.

27. Select the correct statement regarding the recognition and care of cyanosis in newborns.
   A. Cyanosis of the extremities should "pink up" a few minutes after birth.
   B. Cyanosis of the tongue and mucous membranes should "pink up" a few minutes after birth.
   C. Low-concentration O_2 (40% or less) should only be given to newborns in respiratory distress due to the danger of blindness.
   D. The use of cooled O_2 is better for the treatment of cyanosis in a premature baby.

28. Generally, the amniotic sac will break at the beginning of labor. Occasionally, it may encase the baby at delivery. Your care should include:

    A. Rupture of the sac as soon as you observe it in the vaginal opening.
    B. Puncture of the sac as soon as the head is delivered and removal of it from the baby's face.
    C. Transportation of the baby in the sac, as it will only occur in cases of stillborns.
    D. Removal of the cord from around the baby's neck without breaking the sac.

29. During a breech delivery, you should:

    A. Pull the baby's head out after the legs and trunk deliver.
    B. Expect the baby to be born face up.
    C. Transport immediately, as these cases never deliver spontaneously.
    D. Insert a gloved finger in the vagina and keep the walls of the vagina from compressing the baby's airway.

30. Just after your arrival at the scene of an emergency childbirth call, the water breaks and the cord becomes visible outside of the vagina. The woman is crowning, and you should:

    A. Build an oxygen tent around the woman's perineum.
    B. Cover the cord with moist, cool dressings.
    C. Place your gloved hand inside the mother's vagina and push the baby's head up off the cord.
    D. Pull the cord out as far as possible and wrap in sterile aluminum foil.

31. A newborn has just delivered from the birth canal and is breathing. Your initial care for the infant will include:

    A. Immediately drying the infant of amniotic fluid.
    B. Positioning the newborn's head slightly higher than its body.
    C. Positioning the neck in a slightly flexed position.
    D. Suctioning the infant's airway for no less than 10 seconds at a time.

32. When should the Apgar score be calculated for a newborn?

    A. At 1 minute after birth.
    B. At 5 minutes after birth.
    C. At 1 and 5 minutes after birth.
    D. At 5 and 10 minutes after birth.

33. Lisa's newborn has a cardiac rate of less than 100 and a slow respiratory rate. What is the partial Apgar score for Lisa's baby?

    A. 1.
    B. 2.
    C. 3.
    D. 4.

34. Lisa's newborn has fair muscle tone, weak reflex irritability, and is somewhat pink. Her newborn's Apgar score for these three elements is:

    A. 1.
    B. 2.
    C. 3.
    D. 4.

35. About 1 out of every 80 births produces twins. Select the correct statement regarding the delivery of twins.

    A. Twins will always be born with a common placenta.
    B. Twins will always be born with individual placentas.
    C. The umbilical cord should not be cut after the delivery of the first baby.
    D. Twins will usually be born within 45 minutes of each other.

36. A premature infant generally weighs less than 5½ pounds (2.5 kg) or is born before eight months of pregnancy. Select the correct statement regarding the handling of a premature infant.

    A. A premature infant is a mouth breather and must be kept cool to prevent infection.
    B. A premature infant should be kept warm and given oxygen directly by mask at 4 liters per minute.
    C. A premature infant must be kept warm and observed for any bleeding of the umbilical cord.

D. A premature infant should be kept at 100°F. The mouth should be suctioned frequently, because premature infants are primarily mouth breathers.

37. In an ectopic pregnancy, the egg is implanted outside of the uterus. A woman of childbearing age may be suspected of an ectopic pregnancy if her symptoms are:

   A. Warm, dry skin and lack of hunger.
   B. A missed menstrual period and complaints of pain under the diaphragm.
   C. A missed menstrual period and normal blood pressure.
   D. Vaginal spotting and regular menstrual periods.

38. Resuscitation of a newborn should begin if the baby:

   A. Does not begin spontaneous breathing within 30 seconds of delivery.
   B. Has large, multiple blisters on the skin.
   C. Has a foul smell about the body and amniotic fluid.
   D. Has a very soft head.

39. Select the response that lists, in the order of most to least common frequency, the steps in resuscitation of a newborn.

   A. Oxygen, chest compressions, bag-mask ventilation, medications.
   B. Oxygen, tactile stimulation, bag-mask ventilation, chest compressions.
   C. Bag-mask ventilation, chest compression, suction, warming.
   D. Warming, suctioning, oxygen, bag-mask ventilation.

40. You have just assisted in the delivery of a newborn and have placed the infant in a warm environment. You should next assess the infant's:

   A. Respiratory effort.
   B. Heart rate.
   C. Reflex irritability.
   D. Color.

41. After performing the assessment you selected in the previous question, you should next assess the infant's:

   A. Respiratory effort.

B. Heart rate.
C. Reflex irritability.
D. Color.

42. Signs of respiratory distress in the newborn include all of the following except:

    A. Irregular respirations.
    B. Nasal flaring.
    C. Grunting respirations.
    D. Sternal retractions.

43. When performing artificial ventilation on a newborn using a bag-mask device, you should ventilate at a rate of:

    A. 30–40 breaths per minute.
    B. 40–60 breaths per minute.
    C. 50–70 breaths per minute.
    D. 60–80 breaths per minute.

44. Chest compressions should be performed on a newborn if the heart rate is:

    A. Less than 120 beats per minute.
    B. Rapidly increasing from 80 beats per minute.
    C. Greater than 100 beats per minute.
    D. Less than 60 beats per minute.

45. Babies of drug or alcohol addicted mothers will generally exhibit:

    A. High birth weights.
    B. Sedate behavior.
    C. Smaller than normal heads.
    D. Severe respiratory depression.

Answers with Rationale

1. **(B)** Human beings are considered to be infants from birth to age 1. Children are generally 1 to 12 years old. From age 12, persons are considered to be adults.

2. **(B)** Croup, which is an inflammatory condition of the upper airway involving the vocal cords, subglottic tissue, and trachea, generally occurs in children from age six months to three years. Assessment of a croup patient will reveal a runny nose, wheezing, stridor, and a seal-like barking cough. With severe croup, the patient will have nasal flaring, retractions between the ribs, and cyanosis.

3. **(C)** A patient suffering from epiglottitis will have a fever, experience pain swallowing, and have trouble breathing. The patient will often be sitting, leaning forward. Drooling will also be evident. Onset of epiglottitis is usually sudden.

4. **(D)** Croup or acute epiglottitis should be treated with high-concentration O_2, and the patient should be placed in a sitting position. Back blows or chest thrusts will do nothing for these obstructions. Examination of the airway by introduction of a foreign object may precipitate spasms of the larynx.

5. **(B)** The best place to monitor the pulse rate of a neonate is the brachial artery found in the upper arm.

6. **(B)** A tepid (room-temperature) sponge bath can be given to cool a febrile patient found in convulsions. Do not use ice water. Cooling a child to the point of shivering may actually raise the temperature. An oral thermometer should not be used in a convulsing patient of any age. These convulsions usually last only a few minutes.

7. **(B)** Probably the most important action you can take when dealing with an injured child is to communicate on a level he or she can understand. Use of first names is important. A child can handle pain if prepared for it. Keeping the parents close may help relieve some the child's fears. Covering open wounds and splinting will help reduce the child's

fright about injuries. Be sure to show the child that body parts are still there before covering or splinting, as the child may fear a part has been "cut off."

8. (B) An abused child may give several indicators of the condition through his or her behavior. These indicators include a wariness of adult contact, desire to go to school early and return late, desire to avoid going home when it seems appropriate, and exaggerated reactions to the sounds of other children crying.

9. (C) When handling a child you suspect has been abused, report all your findings to the Emergency Department physician receiving the child. Do not criticize the parents or put them "on trial." If the parents refuse consent to transport, you may not do so. Notify the proper authorities in your community of the conditions present at the scene and your examination findings. These authorities could be the police or Children's Services Division of the state's Department of Human Resources.

10. (C) The average vital signs for a 6-year-old child are pulse of 80–100, blood pressure around 100/56, and respirations of 20 to 25 per minute. Answer A shows the vitals for a 1-year-old. Answer B shows the vitals for a 2-year-old. Answer D shows the vitals for a 10-year-old.

11. (B) A blood pressure cuff should cover about two-thirds of the upper arm in any patient situation. A too-small cuff will give erroneously high readings; a too-large cuff will read low. If the BP is taken in the thigh, it should be charted as such.

12. (A) SIDS babies do not die of suffocation from pillows or blankets. The disease is not contagious or hereditary. Generally, CPR will not revive a SIDS baby but will reassure both the parents and rescue personnel that all actions to revive the child have been done.

13. (B) Two-year-old Charlie should be given water to dilute the ferrous sulphate tablets and syrup of ipecac to induce vomiting. Perform this care after contacting either the poison control center or Medical Control.

14. (C) The third stage of labor is from the time the baby is delivered until the placenta is passed. The first stage of labor starts with the beginning

of contractions, often evidenced by a "bloody show." The first stage ends when dilation of the cervix is complete. The second stage of labor begins when the cervix is fully dilated and ends when the baby is born.

15. (C) Guidelines include remaining at the scene if contractions are 2 to 3 minutes apart and last up to 45 seconds each, or if crowning is present. The length of labor of a first-time mother (primigravida) is generally twice that of a woman who has had a baby before (multigravida). If delivery of the placenta takes more than 20 minutes, transport immediately. Should either the mother or baby become distressed, transport or call for a mobile neonatal intensive care unit, if available in your community.

16. (D) Placenta previa is a condition in which the placenta is out of its normal position, having grown over the birth canal. Do not attempt any type of vaginal exam if bleeding is present in a pregnant patient. Transport immediately and treat for shock, as visible blood loss may be minimal. Monitor fetal heart tones. Abruptio placentae is an early separation of the placenta; death of the fetus is likely unless this condition can be corrected in minutes. Eclampsia is a condition of convulsion in the later stages of pregnancy and is often caused by hypertension.

17. (A) A pregnant woman found in convulsions should be treated for the seizure as any other convulsing patient would be. Transportation should be done with the patient on her left side (reduces the weight on the vena cava), with her head elevated 30 to 40 degrees. She is probably experiencing convulsions related to hypertension. Examination of the perineum is not indicated under these stated conditions.

18. (C) Proper care for a pregnant patient who is bleeding heavily from the vagina includes treatment of shock and high-concentration O_2 delivery. Do not pack the vagina with any material. Save all evidence of bleeding to assist the physician in determining the amount of blood loss and possibly finding parts of the placenta. Should the bleeding be mild, transport the woman in a comfortable position, preferably on her left side.

19. (B) If the pregnant woman thinks she is about to deliver, she probably is. If this is her first baby, you probably will have lots of time to transport unless crowning or a desire to move her bowels is present. Back pains are normal during labor. Three-minute intervals for contractions do not generally signal imminent delivery.

Pediatric Emergencies and Childbirth 231

20. (B) The delivery surface should project at least 2 feet past the mother's buttocks to prevent dropping of the newborn and provide a place to put the baby following delivery. The woman's head should be elevated by two or three pillows, and her legs and feet should be well apart. A firm, level surface is most desirable for delivery.

21. (C) As the baby's head begins to push out of the vagina, gently press against the head with the palm of your hand, preventing an explosive birth. Avoid pushing in on the soft areas (fontanelles) of the baby's head, as the brain is just below the skin. The woman should be encouraged to pant during contractions to relieve some of her urge to push. The EMT should avoid touching the mother's vagina in most cases and can check for the presence of the cord around the baby's neck after the head is delivered.

22. (B) When clearing the newborn's airways, first gently suck out the mouth and then the nose. This should be done as soon as possible after the head is delivered. Continue suctioning for no longer than 10 seconds and continuously monitor the heart rate.

23. (A) After the baby has been delivered, immediately place the baby on the table area between the mother's legs and re-suction. Do not place the baby on the mother's abdomen, as this may cause blood loss to the infant as blood flows back down to the placenta. Do not cut the umbilical until the baby is breathing well and the umbilical cord stops pulsing (usually four or five minutes). Don't pick up the baby by the ankles alone, as you may drop him or her.

24. (A) Proper care for the umbilical cord includes double-clamping after pulsations have stopped. Place clamps about midway between the mother and baby, not closer than 6 inches to the baby. Then cut the cord and tie the baby's cord distal to the clamp. Use only sterile umbilical tape to tie the cord. Blood loss from either the baby's umbilical or remaining umbilical of the mother can become fatal rapidly.

25. (C) After the delivery of the placenta, firm massage of the mother's uterus will cause it to contract thereby reducing bleeding. Blood loss in excess of one-half pint is serious and may require treatment for shock. Generally, do not transport until the placenta is delivered, unless bleeding is excessive or 20 minutes has elapsed since the baby's birth. Do not

pack the vagina, even if bleeding is excessive. Cover with sanitary pad and transport.

26. (C) Collect all parts of the afterbirth, as a thorough exam must be done of it to ensure complete passage. Time of birth is recorded for the birth of the baby. After delivery of the placenta, lower the mother's legs to a level position, support them, and cover her vagina with a sanitary pad. If bleeding persists, treat her aggressively for shock and administer high-concentration O_2.

27. (B) Cyanosis of a newborn's tongue and mucous membranes should "pink up" just a few minutes after birth. Cyanosis of the extremities is common in cool babies and may be present for weeks. Newborns in severe respiratory distress should be given high-level O_2 to reduce hypoxia. Warm O_2 is preferable to cool O_2 to prevent cooling of the baby.

28. (B) Rupture the amniotic sac as soon as the baby's head is delivered. Rupture prior to the delivery of the baby's head may cause a prolapsed cord or airway problem for the baby.

29. (D) During a breech delivery, once the baby's hips are delivered, place a gloved finger in the vagina to provide an air passage. Never pull on a baby to speed delivery. A breech baby is generally born face down. Delivery should continue rapidly.

30. (C) In the case of a prolapsed cord and crowning, pushing the baby's head up off the cord may keep the cord from being pinched off. If just the cord is present, cover it with a sterile, moist dressing. Place the mother either on her side in a knee-chest position or on her back with the hips elevated; administer O_2; and transport rapidly.

31. (A) All newborns have difficulty tolerating a cold environment. Heat loss may be prevented by quickly drying the infant and placing the naked infant against the body of the mother, with covers over both. A newborn should be placed on his or her back in a slight Trendelenburg (head down) position with the neck slightly extended. Deep suctioning may produce a vagal response and cause a slowing of the heart rate and/or cessation of breathing; therefore, suctioning should not be continued for more than 10 seconds at a time. Monitor the infant's heart rate while suctioning.

Pediatric Emergencies and Childbirth 233

32. (C) The Apgar score should be calculated at one and five minutes after birth. A score of 8 to 10 can be expected for most newborns after five minutes.

33. (B) The infant's cardiac rate of less than 100 will give the child a score of 1. The infant's slow, shallow, or labored respirations score a 1. Therefore, the partial Apgar score for Lisa's baby is 2. No cardiac output is a 0 and a rate above 100 receives a score of 2.

34. (C) Normal muscle tone is a sign of good oxygenation and would score a 2. This infant is weak and gets a score of 1. When you snap a finger against the sole of the baby's foot, the baby should cry and try to move his foot away. This is normal and scores a 2. A weak cry scores a 1. The feet and lips of a baby should "pink up" within a few minutes of birth for a score of 2. If the body is pink but the feet and lips remain blue, the score is 1. The score of 0 is assigned if the entire baby is pale or blue. Lisa's newborn has a total Apgar score (from questions 33 and 34) of 5.

35. (D) Twins are generally delivered within 45 minutes of one another. They may share a common placenta or each have his or her own. It is extremely important to prevent any bleeding from the umbilical cords in the delivery of twins, as blood loss might be fatal to the second baby sharing a common placenta.

36. (C) Aside from receiving resuscitation, a premature infant must be kept warm and observed for any bleeding of the umbilical cord. A cool baby uses more oxygen. Dry the baby thoroughly; cover all but the face with warmed blankets or aluminum foil to preserve body heat. If possible, keep the baby's environment around 90°F. Oxygen should be given in about 40% concentrations in a tent rather than directly by mask. Premature babies are primarily nose breathers.

37. (B) A woman of childbearing age who has recently missed a menstrual period and complains of pain under the diaphragm, or a tender bloated abdomen, may be suspected of ectopic pregnancy. This patient may show signs of shock if the pregnancy causes a rupture of the fallopian tubes or stomach. Blood pressure may be higher than normal, or low due to shock.

38. **(A)** Resuscitation of a newborn should start if the baby does not begin spontaneous breathing within 30 seconds after delivery. If large, multiple blisters are present on the skin, if the amniotic fluid is foul-smelling, or if the entire head is very soft, the baby is probably dead.

39. **(D)** Most newborns require no resuscitation beyond drying, warming, positioning, suctioning, and tactile stimulation. If the infant does not respond to these steps, reassessment prior to each of the following steps is in order: oxygen therapy, bag-mask ventilation, and chest compression.

40. **(A)** Immediately after delivering a newborn, you should dry and suction the infant and place it in a warm environment. Next, assess the infant's breathing rate and depth, which should increase immediately with brief stimulation. An infant in respiratory distress should not be stimulated more than twice before positive-pressure ventilations are initiated.

41. **(B)** When ventilations are adequate, the heart rate should then be checked. If the infant's heart rate is less than 100 beats per minute, positive-pressure ventilations should be started immediately. If the heart rate is greater than 100 beats per minute and spontaneous respirations are present, the infant's color may be assessed next.

42. **(A)** Irregular respirations are common in newborns. Nasal flaring, grunting respirations, and sternal retractions all indicate respiratory distress.

43. **(B)** Adequate ventilation of the newborn with a bag-mask device should occur with a rate of 40–60 breaths per minute. Normal breathing rates for a newborn are 30–60 breaths per minute. Indications for positive-pressure ventilation include apnea, a heart rate less than 100 beats per minute, and persistent central cyanosis in a maximal oxygen environment. It is best to begin bag-mask ventilations with small volumes, increasing rapidly through small increments, until an adequate tidal volume is achieved. Inability to inflate the lungs adequately requires further suctioning and repositioning of the head. A tight face mask seal must also be maintained.

44. (D) Chest compressions should be performed on a newborn if the heart rate is less than 60 beats per minute or 60–80 beats per minute and not rapidly increasing despite adequate ventilations with 100% oxygen for approximately 30 seconds. Compressions should be performed at a rate of 100–120 times per minute accompanied by positive-pressure ventilations with 100% O_2 at a rate of 40–60 per minute.

45. (D) Babies born of drug-addicted mothers or suffering from fetal alcohol syndrome are usually premature, have low birth weight, are irritable, and suffer severe respiratory depression. Personal protection, as always, is important because the mother and baby may be HVB or HIV infected.

12 Environmental Injury Emergencies

This chapter focuses on common environmental emergencies, including such topics as thermal and chemical burns, exposure to cold and hypothermia, toxic gases, and radioactive materials. There are questions on response to the scene, EMT protective measures, patient assessment, and patient care. Questions dealing with heat exhaustion and heat stroke, along with some questions on water hazards and scuba diving maladies, are also included.

    You can anticipate several test questions on state and national certification examinations regarding the subject matter contained in this chapter.

1. Immediate care for burns caused by a liquid chemical includes:

   A. Irrigation after the clothing has been removed.
   B. Use of a powerful stream of water to irrigate burned tissue.
   C. Use of a garden hose to irrigate large affected areas.
   D. Use of neutralizing solution prior to irrigation with water.

2. Proper emergency care for chemical burns to the eyes includes:

   A. Irrigating alkali burns for up to 20 minutes.
   B. Irrigating acid burns for up to 20 minutes.
   C. Irrigating alkali burns with a mixture of vinegar and water.
   D. Irrigating alkali burns with baking soda.

3. During your assessment and care of a patient with an electrical burn, you should:

   A. Cover the burns with moist, sterile dressings.
   B. Examine for entrance and exit wounds.
   C. Be prepared to administer chest compressions, as cardiac arrest often occurs in such a patient without respiratory arrest.
   D. Immerse the burn area in ice water to reduce deep tissue burning.

4. Characteristics of a second-degree burn include:

   A. Reddening of the skin.
   B. Damage to but not through the epidermis, with resultant blisters.
   C. Damage to but not through the dermis, with resultant blisters.
   D. Damage to and including the subcutaneous layer, appearing white or brown in color.

5. Thirty-year-old Jim Brown has burns on the front and back of both his legs and arms. Approximately what percentage of his body has been involved?

   A. 27%.
   B. 36%.
   C. 45%.
   D. 54%.

6. Four-year-old Chris Brown has been pulled from the same fire in which his father was involved. He has burns on his head and back.

What approximate percentage of the child's body surface has been burned?

A. 18%.
B. 27%.
C. 36%.
D. 45%.

7. Called to assist at the scene of a kitchen fire, you find 19-year-old Rose has burned both of her arms while trying to put out a grease fire. She has reddening and blisters on each arm. You should:

   A. Cover her arms with dry, sterile dressings.
   B. Immerse her arms in cold water for at least 10 minutes before dressing.
   C. Apply copious amounts of petroleum jelly to relieve pain.
   D. Apply silver nitrate to her burns, cover with sterile dressings, and transport.

8. Allen Martin was filling the gas tank on his lawn mower when it suddenly burst into flames. Mr. Martin quickly threw the gas can away from himself. Mr. Martin's voice is hoarse, the hairs in his nostrils are singed, his face is blistered, and both arms are reddened. You should classify his burns as:

   A. Critical.
   B. Severe.
   C. Moderate.
   D. Minor.

9. Your care for an unconscious MVA patient with second- and third-degree burns over 45% of the body should include:

   A. Immobilizing the spine.
   B. Applying ice packs on extremities.
   C. Covering eyes with dry, sterile dressings.
   D. Administering nonhumidified O_2.

10. Care for a patient with second- and third-degree burns on both of her arms should include:

    A. Frequently monitoring distal pulse.
    B. Skipping the taking of blood pressure.

C. Avoiding monitoring the radial pulse.
D. Applying silver nitrate and burn dressings.

11. From the burn patients below, select the one you should transport to a burn center first.

    A. 81% third-degree.
    B. 60% without pain.
    C. 60% with pain.
    D. 45% circumferential burns of the chest.

12. Heat exhaustion typically presents with:

    A. Weakness, dizziness, and cool skin.
    B. Weakness and flushed, hot skin.
    C. Muscle cramps, wet skin, and thirst.
    D. Dizziness and hot, dry skin.

13. Choose the group of signs and symptoms that best describes the condition of a person experiencing heat stroke.

    A. Pale, moist skin; rapid pulse; and slow, deep respirations.
    B. Hot, dry skin; rapid pulse; and slow, deep respirations.
    C. Hot, dry skin; normal pulse; and normal respirations.
    D. Pale, moist skin; weak pulse; and rapid respirations.

14. Care for a patient suspected of heat stroke (core temp. 106°F) should include:

    A. Immersing the patient in water approximately 41°C in temperature.
    B. Covering the patient with blankets.
    C. Covering the patient with wet sheets.
    D. Administering large quantities of water and salt tablets.

15. While fighting a brush fire, Todd Unger experiences painful muscle spasms of the arms and legs. Your care for Mr. Unger should be to administer:

    A. Salt tablets and water.
    B. Many glasses of cold water.
    C. Six salt tablets and one glass of ice water.
    D. Vigorous massage to his arms and legs to increase circulation.

16. Select the correct statement regarding body temperature and its maintenance.

    A. A human cannot survive body-core temperatures higher than 105°F or lower than 90°F.
    B. Shivering is an activity that reduces body heat by causing the vessels of the skin to dilate.
    C. Evaporation causes body heat to rise.
    D. Respiration exhausts much body heat.

17. You are called to treat Roy, a 32-year-old male jogger. He is unconscious, hot to the touch, and has dry skin. You suspect:

    A. Heat exhaustion.
    B. Heat cramps.
    C. Heat stroke.
    D. Heat hyperventilation syndrome.

18. Proper care for frostbitten extremities includes:

    A. Gentle rubbing with snow to increase peripheral circulation.
    B. Warm-water immersion, with water temperature between 115°F and 120°F.
    C. Protection from further damage by moving the patient to a warmer environment and transporting to a hospital for rewarming.
    D. Rapid rewarming in room air or warm water at less than 112°F.

19. Proper transportation care of a frostbitten patient includes:

    A. Elevating thawed extremities.
    B. Lowering thawed extremities.
    C. Wrapping affected extremities in sterile, dry dressings and transporting with those extremities lower than the level of the heart.
    D. Allowing the patient to walk to the ambulance to increase circulation in thawed feet and legs.

20. Systemic hypothermia is said to have occurred when the:

    A. Body is unable to rewarm itself.
    B. Body-core temperature falls below 85°F.
    C. Body begins to shiver.
    D. Body temperature falls below 90°F.

21. Lacking a thermometer, estimate the body temperature of a person suffering from hypothermia who is displaying signs of lethargy, sleepiness, and confusion.

    A. 90°F to 95°F.
    B. 86°F to 90°F.
    C. 80°F to 86°F.
    D. Below 80°F.

22. Typically, the cause of death for a person who has suffered hypothermia is:

    A. Respiratory arrest.
    B. Ventricular fibrillation.
    C. Pulmonary edema.
    D. Central nervous system standstill.

23. The proper care for a person suffering severe hypothermia would be to:

    A. Warm rapidly by use of heating pads or warm-water immersion.
    B. Administer high-concentration O_2 from an O_2 tank packed in ice.
    C. Stabilize temperature but do not attempt rewarming.
    D. Vigorously attempt to rewarm by rubbing all of the extremities with warm, moist washcloths.

24. What is the most penetrating type of nuclear radiation?

    A. Alpha.
    B. Beta.
    C. Gamma.
    D. Neutron.

25. Select the correct statement regarding the emergency care of a patient who has been exposed to nuclear radiation.

    A. A patient who has received a whole external body dose of radiation presents a danger to the care provider.
    B. A patient who has inhaled or swallowed radioactive material poses a great threat to the people caring for the patient.
    C. Radioactive materials on the skin or clothing prohibit any emergency medical care prior to decontamination.
    D. A patient's nasal passages should be swabbed and swabs saved if inhalation of radioactive smoke or particles is suspected.

26. Called to a MVA, you discover that a semi-truck displaying a radioactive warning placard has been involved. A liquid spill has occurred. The driver of the truck is in the cab and appears unconscious. You should:

    A. Immediately extricate the driver and immobilize his spine prior to moving.
    B. Call the fire department and request a Geiger counter before approaching the truck.
    C. Place plastic bags on your boots and effect rapid extrication to an area away from the truck.
    D. Approach this scene as any other, since there is no chance for radioactive contamination because the leaking material is a liquid.

27. Choose the correct statement regarding electrical hazards.

    A. High voltage lines are rubber-insulated wires.
    B. Ordinary house current cannot harm you unless your feet are wet.
    C. The human body is an excellent conductor.
    D. Current will not flow through the body unless both ends of a fallen live wire are touched.

28. Select the answer that best states conditions or effects of near-drowning.

    A. Destruction of blood cells (hemolysis) occurs most often in salt-water drownings.
    B. Pulmonary edema is most severe from fresh-water near-drownings.
    C. The lungs frequently fill with water in near-drownings, making ventilation very difficult.
    D. Artificial ventilations may become easier after the patient has been unconscious for a short period of time.

29. Dispatched to a swimming center where an all-city swim meet is in progress, you find lifeguards performing artificial ventilations on a 19-year-old male. The lifeguards explain that he suddenly stopped in the middle of his third lap and sank. You should suspect:

    A. Immersion hypothermia.
    B. Heat exhaustion.
    C. Breath-holding blackout.
    D. Swimmer's ear.

30. Called to a small bay just north of the city limits, you find a scuba-diving student lying on the ground complaining of sharp pains in his ears, and vertigo. You should suspect:

    A. "Squeeze" injury caused by rapid descent.
    B. "The bends," or decompression sickness.
    C. Air embolism affecting the brain.
    D. Nitrogen narcosis.

31. At the scene of another scuba-diving accident, the diver's buddy explains that the female patient made a rapid ascent. The patient complains of chest pain, blurred vision, and pain in leg muscles and abdomen. Your care for this patient should include:

    A. Administering low-concentration O_2.
    B. Placing the patient in a sitting position with her head elevated.
    C. Treating for shock by raising her feet slightly.
    D. Placing the patient on her left side with her head and chest down.

32. The "Lund and Browder" chart is used in calculating:

    A. Scuba-diving bottom times.
    B. Electrical energy estimates from burns.
    C. Rewarming times for hypothermia.
    D. Thermal burn surface area percentages.

33. When attempting to rewarm a hypothermic patient, you should be aware that:

    A. Ventricular fibrillation is more easily converted in a cold patient.
    B. Rewarming can cause death.
    C. Warm-water immersion must be done in water 115°F or warmer.
    D. A breeze will increase the speed of rewarming.

34. When examining a 3-year-old child for burns, you should suspect possible child abuse if:

    A. One foot is burned by hot water.
    B. One palm is burned by flame.
    C. Several cigarette burns are present.
    D. The child's buttocks, legs, and lower trunk are burned.

35. Called to a golf course during an electrical storm, you find an unconscious male who has been hit by lightning. You should:

A. Start CPR even after 30 minutes have passed, as this patient is an exception to the 6 to 10 minute rule.
B. Start CPR if needed unless entrance and exit wounds are present, in which case the patient cannot be resuscitated.
C. Not touch the patient for at least 6 minutes because his body contains electrical current.
D. Hyperextend his neck to open the airway.

36. The most important fact you should keep in mind while delivering care to a person with a lowered body temperature is that:

    A. Resuscitation can be successful after long periods of apparent cardiac arrest.
    B. Rewarming can be done only in a hospital setting.
    C. Most body heat loss is from respiration.
    D. Exposure to cold air is more dangerous than exposure to cold water.

37. All pulseless, nonbreathing patients submerged in water less than _____ should be resuscitated.

    A. 90°F.
    B. 85°F.
    C. 80°F.
    D. 70°F.

38. When called to an accident scene involving a spill of hazardous materials, you should first:

    A. Approach from upwind.
    B. Notify CHEMTREC.
    C. Identify the exact material spilled.
    D. Do a complete examination on your patient before moving him in case there are fractures present.

39. You are on the first unit to arrive at the scene of a two-vehicle MVA. As you approach you notice an orange hazardous material placard on the side of a delivery van but you are unable to read the figures on the placard. What does an orange background color signify?

    A. Poisonous material.
    B. Corrosive material.
    C. Flammable material.
    D. Explosive material.

40. While the process of identifying a hazardous material is being conducted, you should:

    A. Seek protection in low-lying areas.
    B. Avoid conversation with company safety officers until the victims are removed from the hazardous area.
    C. Establish a hazard zone.
    D. Limit access to the immediate area of the hazard to only one EMT.

41. Decontamination of a patient exposed to a hazardous material should be conducted:

    A. At the hospital.
    B. Prior to any medical treatment being rendered.
    C. In the ambulance.
    D. Prior to transportation.

42. You are called to a MVA and discover that a transport truck with a visible vapor cloud is involved. You determine from the warning placard that the truck is transporting liquid methane. You should:

    A. Attempt to extinguish any fire.
    B. Set flares at 1500 feet distance.
    C. Evacuate upwind bystanders.
    D. Avoid breathing vapors.

Answers with Rationale

1. **(C)** Immediate care for almost all liquid chemical burns should be irrigation with water. Irrigation should be done as soon as possible, with clothing removed after irrigation of the area has begun. Be sure to remove the patient's footgear since the chemical will pool there. Burned tissue is delicate, and powerful streams of water could cause tearing of the skin. Do not attempt to neutralize chemicals prior to copious water irrigation.

2. **(A)** Alkali burns to the eyes should be irrigated for at least 20 minutes. If in doubt of the chemical, use 20 minutes as a rule of thumb. Never use a neutralizing agent in the eyes. Avoid a direct irrigation stream on the cornea, but rather wash from medial to lateral. Acid burns require about 5 minutes of irrigation. After irrigation, cover both eyes with moist, sterile dressings, and transport.

3. **(B)** During your assessment of a patient with an electrical burn, first care for the ABCs of airway, breathing, and circulation; then examine for both entrance and exit burns, which are typically in the hands and feet. Remove shoes and socks for examination. Ventilatory arrest is a common occurrence. Cardiac dysrhythmias may cause cardiac arrest. Dry, sterile dressings are indicated for electrical burns.

4. **(C)** A second-degree burn includes damage to the epidermis and dermis and often results in blisters. This burn does not damage tissue below the dermis. A first-degree burn appears as reddening of the skin. A third-degree burn involves tissue below the dermis and may appear white or charred.

5. **(D)** Mr. Brown's burns cover approximately 54% of his body surface. Each arm is 9% (18%) and each leg is 18% (36%).

6. **(C)** Chris Brown has burns involving his head (18%) and back (18%), for a total of 36% body surface involvement. The head of a small child represents a much larger surface than an adult's head; therefore, it is considered 18% instead of 9%.

7. (A) Rose has first- and second-degree burns on both arms. The rule of cooling may apply if a burn is less than 10% of the body surface. Rose has 18% involvement. If the skin or clothing is still hot, cooling is in order. She can be transported with her arms dressed in dry, sterile dressings.

8. (A) Mr. Martin's burn injury would be classified as critical. He shows signs of respiratory involvement, as his voice is hoarse and the hairs in his nostrils are singed. He has second-degree burns on his face and first-degree on his arms.

9. (A) Care for a MVA patient with major burns should include spinal immobilization first. Often the EMT will overlook this type of emergency medical care because of the presence of other major trauma. Ice packs may cause further damage to skin and underlying tissue and should be avoided. Eyes should be covered with moist, sterile dressings. Humidified O_2 should be given in high concentrations. A burn sheet is indicated.

10. (A) Burns on extremities can cause severe swelling, leading to limited or complete occlusion of distal circulation. Distal pulses must be monitored frequently. The blood pressure cuff should be applied to nonaffected extremities. Silver nitrate should not be applied in the field.

11. (D) The burn patient with circumferential burns on the chest should be transported first, as swelling may reduce chest wall movement to a point of inadequate ventilation. The next patient to transport should be the 60% burn without pain. The third one is 60% with pain. The 81% burn patient will probably not survive and should be transported only after the others have received care.

12. (A) Heat exhaustion typically presents with the patient complaining of weakness or dizziness. The skin is cool and wet. Heat stroke presents with hot, often dry skin and body weakness, rapidly progressing to unconsciousness.

13. (B) A person experiencing heat stroke will most likely have hot, dry skin; a rapid pulse; and slow, deep respirations.

14. (C) Care for heat stroke requires rapid lowering of the body's temperature to near normal. This can be accomplished by fanning, applying

moist towels, or wrapping the patient in wet sheets. Cold water may be given to a conscious patient. This is a complex medical emergency. Salt tablets will not be of great value. Immersion in icy water may be performed in the E.D. A temperature of 106°F is equal to 41°C.

15. (B) Todd Unger is experiencing heat cramps. Many glasses of cool water should help relieve the spasms as the body's balance is returned. Administering large quantities of salt may actually complicate the problem, as water migrates to salt. Massage of the limbs will be of little use.

16. (D) Respiration exhausts much body heat by blowing off warmed air. Although it is unsafe, the body can survive temperatures in excess of 105°F and lower than 90°F. Evaporation of sweat causes cooling. Shivering is an activity that warms the body.

17. (C) Roy's hot, dry skin should alert you to the possibility that he is suffering a heat stroke. His skin would be wet and near normal temperature if he were suffering heat exhaustion.

18. (C) Proper care of frostbitten extremities is best performed in a controlled environment by medical staff trained to evaluate and treat such cases. Do not rub frostbitten or frozen areas, as this will increase tissue damage.

19. (A) Elevation of thawed extremities is indicated during transportation in order to reduce swelling. The affected areas should be wrapped in loose, dry, sterile dressings. Once an extremity is rewarmed, do not allow any use of the extremity, as the tissue is very delicate and sensitive. Prevent refreezing.

20. (A) Systemic hypothermia is said to have occurred when the body can no longer rewarm itself. This occurs when the body temperature lowers past the point of shivering, which is a rewarming mechanism. Shivering will cease at about 95°F. Hypothermia can occur in environmental temperatures above freezing if the person is not adequately protected from cold, moisture, and wind.

21. (C) Signs of lethargy, sleepiness, and confusion will be present as body-core temperatures lower to the range of 86° to 80°F. Core temperatures between about 86° and 90°F will produce difficulty in speaking,

stumbling, and inability to use hands. Unconsciousness will occur below 80°F.

22. (B) Ventricular fibrillation is typically the cause of death of patients with hypothermia and is caused by cold blood irritating the heart. Such patients are extremely difficult to cardiovert electrically with the use of a defibrillator. They may go into ventricular fibrillation with any sudden jolt or movement.

23. (C) From the choices offered, the most appropriate care for severe hypothermia would be to stabilize the body temperature but not rewarm. Rapid rewarming by use of heating pads and warm-water immersion allows cold blood to reach the heart. Rewarming needs to be done internally (core) to ensure that blood returning from the extremities is warmed prior to reaching the heart. Warm O_2 is indicated to aid in internal warming of blood as it passes through the lungs.

24. (C) Gamma rays will penetrate a body that is not protected by a heavy material, such as lead. Alpha rays can be reflected by light protection, such as a newspaper. Beta rays can be reflected by several layers of clothing. Neutron rays are generally found only at sites with large amounts of radiation, such as a nuclear reactor system.

25. (D) If a patient is suspected of having inhaled radioactive smoke or dust, swab the nasal passages, and save the swabs for later evaluation. This is the best way to determine if contamination of the air passages has occurred. Lifesaving care should be administered before decontamination, when possible. Once a patient has inhaled or swallowed radioactive material, he or she poses little threat to others. The same is true of a large dose by direct exposure. It is the source of radiation from which you must protect yourself.

26. (C) If you suspect radioactive contaminants are present, protect your feet from contaminants with plastic bags and rapidly remove the truck driver from the area. Removal should be to a place that is protected by a mass (ditch, concrete barrier, behind other vehicles, etc.). This area should be upwind from the suspected leak. This patient should be moved rapidly, as if he were in a structural fire, to minimize exposure time.

27. (C) The human body is an excellent conductor of electricity. High-voltage power lines are not insulated by protective rubber. Ordinary house current can cause death if a circuit is completed. Current will flow from a live wire without a broken end being connected (AC current).

28. (D) Artificial ventilations may become easier after a patient has been unconscious for a period of time. Spasms of the larynx will diminish as the patient becomes more hypoxic. Hemolysis occurs most often in fresh-water drownings, as the water enters the more salty blood cells. Pulmonary edema occurs in salt-water drownings, as the lungs become congested from the body fluids joining the salt water in the lungs. It also occurs in fresh-water drownings due to surfactant breakdown and fluid passage into the lungs. Water in the lungs is a problem that does occur at times, but your resuscitation efforts must be continued.

29. (C) He probably experienced a breath-holding blackout. This is common for a person trying to increase time underwater by hyperventilation. The respiratory drive is temporarily overcome, but the patient still needs air. Immersion hypothermia is not likely, nor is heat exhaustion. Swimmer's ear is a condition that usually causes a severe itch in the ear.

30. (A) The scuba-diving student with sharp pains in his ears and with vertigo has probably experienced a "squeeze" injury. This is most often seen when a diver makes a rapid descent without clearing the ears and mask. There may be a print of the mask on the patient's face. The condition can also be caused by ascent, but it is unlikely. Nitrogen narcosis is a "bottom" problem. As the diver ascends, narcosis quickly clears.

31. (D) The symptoms that this scuba diver presents are typical of an air embolism. The patient should be placed on her left side, with her head and chest lower than the trunk and legs. This will help trap air emboli and keep them from migrating to the brain. High-concentration O_2 is also indicated.

32. (D) The "Lund and Browder" chart was developed to determine the percentage of body surface involved in burns. It is extremely useful in the treatment of children.

33. (B) Rewarming of a hypothermic patient can cause death if not done properly. Rewarming can be accomplished by warm-water immersion,

with the water temperature between 100°F and 105°F. A breeze will cool the patient further. Ventricular fibrillation is not easily converted in a hypothermic patient. Some experts prefer to keep the severely hypothermic patient cool until he or she can be effectively treated in the Emergency Department. CPR may not even be ordered by Medical Control until rewarming takes place.

34. (C) Abuse must be suspected in either an adult or a child if several cigarette burns are present. Other signs of child abuse might be both palms burned by flame or both feet equally burned from hot water, causing a burn often resembling a stocking line. If the buttocks, legs, and lower trunk are burned, the child may have been placed in a hot bathtub, most likely by accident.

35. (A) Start CPR on the golfer. Brain death seems to take much longer in patients who are struck by lightning. The patient poses no danger to anyone else. Treat burn wounds with sterile dressings, using moist dressing if burns are still hot to touch. Do not hyperextend the neck, as spinal injury is common in cases of lightning contact.

36. (A) Whether a person is suffering from severe hypothermia from exposure to cold or to cold-water immersion, remember that this patient can survive with a lower body temperature. Aggressive CPR may save a patient thought to be in arrest for many hours. Rewarming is generally not attempted outside the hospital setting. Water conducts heat about 25 times faster than air. Hypothermia may present rapidly in cold-water immersion. Although some body heat is lost from respiration, the majority is lost through the skin.

37. (D) All pulseless, nonbreathing patients submerged in water less than 70°F (21.1°C) should be resuscitated.

38. (A) Approach any scene involving a spill of hazardous material from upwind. Avoid low-lying areas, as toxic or flammable fumes may settle there. CHEMTREC (U.S.A. 1-800-424-9300) (Canada—call CANUTEC 613-966-6666) can be called for advice if you know the nature of the spilled material. You can identify chemicals by reading the placard displayed on the sides of a transporting vehicle. When in doubt, approach with full protective gear (turnouts, airpacks, etc.) and rapidly remove the patient to a safe area.

39. **(D)** The orange background color of the placard alerts you that the material being transported is considered explosive. A white background is used for poisonous materials, and white over black for corrosive materials. Red backgrounds are used to identify flammable materials, and yellow for oxidizers.

40. **(C)** While the process of identifying a hazardous material is going on, a hazard zone should be established. The Hazmat Rule of Thumb is one method of determining the area to be avoided. This method calls for the EMT to hold his arm out straight with the thumb up. The thumb is then centered over the hazardous area. If hazardous material can still be seen, the EMT is too close and the zone should be enlarged. Company safety officers may be able to offer valuable assistance and rescuers should follow their direction. Rescuers should remain upwind of the hazard and avoid low areas where toxic fumes may settle.

41. **(D)** Decontamination of the patient should begin as soon as possible. The patient's clothing should be removed and placed in sealed containers to avoid further spread of the hazardous material. Decontamination of the EMT's clothing and equipment is also important. Continued exposure in a confined area such as the ambulance could adversely affect personnel including those not directly involved in the initial rescue effort. Life threatening conditions can be treated while decontamination procedures are being performed.

42. **(D)** Avoid breathing the vapors of any leaking hazardous material. Request assistance from available hazardous materials team since these incidents are extremely complex in nature. A leaking methane gas fire would not be extinguished unless the flow of the leak could be stopped. If a leaking material is not on fire, attempt to extinguish any possible source of ignition. Always stay upwind of leaks.

13 Behavioral Problems

Although often underemphasized in many EMT courses, mental health problems are frequently encountered by the EMT. Patients who are senile or suicidal can endanger other people while threatening their own lives. Mentally deranged individuals who are potentially violent can be dangerous to the community as a whole. Questions relating to special problems caused by alcohol, hallucinogens, stimulants, and depressants are also included in this chapter.

1. The most commonly abused drug in the United States is:

   A. Cocaine.
   B. Marijuana.
   C. Valium.
   D. Alcohol.

2. Which of the following drugs is considered a hallucinogen?

   A. Seconal.
   B. PCP.
   C. Quaalude.
   D. Valium.

3. Typically, withdrawal from drugs of the stimulant category (amphetamines) will cause:

   A. Increased blood pressure.
   B. Rapid breathing.
   C. Depression.
   D. Sleeplessness.

4. Which of the following drugs is considered a stimulant?

   A. Methadone.
   B. Codeine.
   C. Cocaine.
   D. Heroin.

5. Which of the following drugs is considered a relaxant?

   A. Miltown.
   B. Noludar.
   C. Nembutal.
   D. Marijuana.

6. The most serious symptom of a Crack overdose is:

   A. Chest pain.
   B. Tremors.
   C. Anxiety.
   D. Disorientation.

7. Care for a drug overdose patient includes basic life support (airway maintenance). It is also very important to:

   A. Maintain the patient's consciousness by constant stimulation.
   B. Induce vomiting in all OD cases involving ingested drugs.
   C. Use restraints on hallucinogenic drug patients.
   D. Wear a disposable mask when dealing with drug overdose patients suspected of using injectable drugs such as morphine.

8. The cause of death in depressant drug overdose cases is generally:

   A. Respiratory collapse.
   B. Circulatory collapse.
   C. Stroke.
   D. Vasodilation.

9. Occasionally, a drug addict will try to "kick" the habit. While doing so, he or she may experience drug withdrawal. Symptoms commonly associated with drug withdrawal include:

   A. Hunger.
   B. Intense thirst.
   C. Dry, warm skin.
   D. Seizures.

10. Select the correct statement regarding alcohol withdrawal.

    A. Delirium tremens cases have a high mortality rate.
    B. Alcoholic hallucination without delirium tremens is a sign of impending death.
    C. Onset of delirium tremens usually occurs 8 days after alcohol is withheld from the patient.
    D. Death from delirium tremens is usually caused by respiratory collapse.

11. Inhaled solvents (glue, nail polish, typewriter correction fluid) cause effects similar to those of:

    A. Stimulants.
    B. Alcohol.
    C. Hallucinogens.
    D. Narcotics.

12. A drug that causes "pin-point" pupils is:

    A. Miltown.
    B. Demerol.
    C. Phenobarbital.
    D. Benzedrine.

13. Proper care for an acutely agitated, irrational, or combative patient should include:

    A. Letting the patient sit with the driver so he can see that he is going to a hospital, not a police station.
    B. Using restraints routinely to protect the patient and others.
    C. Allowing the patient to sit unrestrained in the back of the ambulance.
    D. Turning over all such patients to police authorities for transportation.

14. Called to the home of an elderly couple by the wife, you find her husband acting unruly, throwing lamps about, and swearing. He has obviously voided in his pants. Your care for this patient should include:

    A. Immediately restraining his extremities and transporting him.
    B. Reassuring the wife that her husband is ill and is not in control of his mental processes.
    C. Contacting the Emergency Department and advising them that the patient has had a stroke so you can transport.
    D. Asking the wife to remain in the room with you as you try to comfort the patient.

15. When dealing with an emotionally disturbed patient who is menacing a member of his family with a knife, you should:

    A. Ask the family member to remain with you so you can talk the patient down.
    B. Attempt to remove the knife from the patient.
    C. Encourage the family to call the police.
    D. Notify your dispatcher of the need for police backup.

16. Called to a home, you find a 53-year-old female acting irrationally, throwing dishes and glasses against the kitchen wall. Her husband wants her "taken someplace where she won't hurt anyone." After you

try to calm her down and suggest that she needs to go to the hospital, she continues to refuse your help. Generally, you should:

A. Transport her as her husband has authorized.
B. Transport her if the Medical Control physician instructs you to do so.
C. Transport her if the police direct you to do so.
D. Refuse to transport her after the police direct you to do so, as she is now in their custody.

17. General guidelines for the care of a suicidal crisis include:

    A. Remaining open, sympathetic, and professional.
    B. Leaving the patient to call the crisis clinic once you have calmed him or her down.
    C. Being verbally aggressive to an abusive patient, demonstrating to the patient who is in control.
    D. Not directly stating the truth to the patient to buy time until the police arrive.

18. When dispatched to an apartment complex for a "man down, unknown cause," you should:

    A. Wait for police backup.
    B. Cautiously approach the scene and listen for clues of danger.
    C. Request an engine company assist.
    D. Immediately care for the injured party, even if an assailant is present.

19. A rural volunteer ambulance is summoned to a home where a 24-year-old male is threatening suicide. Police backup will not be available for nearly 45 minutes. From inside a locked bedroom, the man states, "I'm going to shoot myself." You should:

    A. Avoid the use of the word "suicide," as this may encourage him to shoot himself.
    B. Determine if he has a plan of action and if he has a gun and bullets.
    C. Attempt to gain access by breaking the door open while your partner goes through a window.
    D. Determine if he has tried suicide before, since statistics show he will not attempt suicide if he has tried it before.

20. Proper management guidelines for a violent patient include:

    A. Approaching him head-on so he isn't threatened.
    B. Telling the patient to "grow up" or "act your age" to bring him back to reality.
    C. Advising the patient that you are not going to stand for his verbal abuse.
    D. Leaving yourself an escape route in case the patient goes "out of control."

21. Management guidelines for the care of a paranoid patient include:

    A. Not looking at the patient because he or she will think you are staring.
    B. Interviewing available family and friends in the patient's presence.
    C. Taking the side of the patient by saying, "Yes, I too am afraid of those people."
    D. Being sneaky and tricking the patient into the ambulance, since you will probably not be able to talk him or her into entering it.

22. Which of the following drugs produces euphoria, drowsiness, insensitivity to pain, nausea, watery eyes, and runny nose?

    A. Cocaine.
    B. Heroin.
    C. Methamphetamine.
    D. Marijuana.

23. Proper care for a phencyclidine (PCP) patient should include:

    A. Talking the patient down from the trip.
    B. Keeping the patient in bright lighting to alleviate fear.
    C. Keeping outside stimulation (lights, noises, etc.) to a minimum.
    D. Talking loudly and clearly, as the patient has difficulty in hearing.

24. Proper care for an intoxicated patient includes:

    A. Administration of aspirin.
    B. Administration of ipecac.
    C. Determination that no other medical problems are present.
    D. Administration of Antabuse.

25. At the scene of a MVA, you observe that an apparently uninjured driver of one of the involved vehicles has slight euphoria, watery eyes, and a runny nose. You might also find that this person has:

   A. Hypotensive blood pressure.
   B. Slow pulse rate.
   C. Slow respiratory rate.
   D. Dilated pupils.

26. When dealing with family members of a deceased patient, you should:

   A. Prevent any of them from reacting strongly and disturbing the others.
   B. Allow the family to be with the deceased.
   C. Administer O_2 to anyone who is crying hysterically.
   D. Wait for the police to arrive, and let them advise the family of the death.

Answers with Rationale

1. (D) The most commonly abused drug in the United States is alcohol.

2. (B) Phencyclidine (PCP), dimethorymethylamphetamine (STP), and D-Lysergic acid diethylamide (LSD) are all considered hallucinogens. Seconal, Quaaludes, and Valium are depressants.

3. (C) Typically, withdrawal from drugs of the stimulant category causes depression, coma, or death. Ingestion of amphetamines generally increases heart rate and blood pressure and may also cause jitters, sleeplessness, and headaches.

4. (C) Cocaine is considered a stimulant and is referred to by several "street names," such as blow, candy, flake, snow, and toot. Codeine, heroin, and methadone are classified as narcotics.

5. (D) Marijuana is classified as a relaxant while Miltown, Noludar, and Nembutal are classified as sedatives and hypnotics.

6. (A) The major threat of Crack overdose is to the cardiopulmonary system. Vasospasm, including intense coronary artery vasoconstriction, causes myocardial ischemia and arterial hypertension and can precipitate a myocardial infarction. Care for a Crack overdose patient includes airway care and evaluation of all major pulses and blood pressure monitoring in each arm since acute increases in blood pressure can lead to aortic dissection. Anxiety, disorientation, and tremors are other signs associated with Crack overdose.

7. (A) It is important to maintain the drug overdose patient's consciousness at all times, as respiratory depression rapidly follows unconsciousness. This can be done by constant stimulation, including talking, gentle shaking, and pinching. Induction of vomiting in a semi-conscious or comatose patient would compromise the patient's airway. Unless a hallucinating patient is a danger to himself or others, avoid the use of restraints, as this action may compound problems. Hepatitis and AIDS can be passed by contact with the patient's fecal material, semen, or blood.

8. (A) The general cause of death from depressant drug overdose is respiratory collapse. Airway care and artificial ventilation are commonly required for such patients.

9. (D) Symptoms commonly associated with drug withdrawal include seizures, diaphoresis, nausea, and vomiting. The patient may also demonstrate signs of nystagmus (a constant, involuntary, cyclical movement of the eyeball, which can be in any direction).

10. (A) Delirium tremens cases have a high rate of mortality. This is a true medical emergency. Alcohol hallucinations may precede DTs or may occur alone. Alcohol hallucinations are not a sign of impending death even though the patient may believe they are. Delirium tremens usually occurs from one to seven days after a chronic alcoholic ceases ingestion of the drug. Death from DTs is caused by many body imbalances, loss of fluids, and shock.

11. (B) Inhaled solvents cause effects similar to alcohol ingestion.

12. (B) Narcotic drugs such as opium, heroin, codeine, and Demerol cause "pin-point" pupils. Miltown and phenobarbital are depressants and will probably cause pupils to dilate. Benzedrine will also cause dilated pupils.

13. (C) Unless you truly feel the patient is a danger to himself or others, he should be allowed to sit unrestrained in the back of the ambulance. The patient should not be allowed to sit in the driver's compartment, because he might experience a sudden change of mood and become violent. Many times, the police will request the ambulance service to transport such patients. This is a medical problem, and these patients require professional evaluation and care.

14. (B) In the case of the unruly husband, you may suspect senile dementia. Reassurance of the wife is indicated. The elderly husband is not in control of his mental processes. If the patient is expressing anger toward his wife, remove her to another room. Your best action would be to try to talk the patient back to reality and avoid the use of restraints. This patient needs to be seen in the Emergency Department but should not be taken against his will, unless the police authorize you to do so.

15. (D) When dealing with an emotionally disturbed patient who is menacing, notify your dispatcher of the situation and the need for police assistance. The EMT should initiate this call to avoid making the family feel guilty. If there is an argument between a family member and the patient, separate the parties, preferably by removing one to another room to lessen the already existing tensions. Do not take sides in the argument. Do not try to physically disarm the patient, but do attempt to talk him into placing the weapon on a chair or floor. Make sure to situate yourself between the weapon and the patient before proceeding with your care. Always keep the patient's hands in sight. Do not approach him if you cannot be certain he is totally unarmed.

16. (C) The woman in this situation should be transported only if the police direct you to do so. The police can also transport if not medically contraindicated. Legally, her husband is not her guardian unless appointed by the court. The physician at Medical Control cannot order her to be transported either. This problem is not uncommon.

17. (A) The EMT must remain open, sympathetic, and professional during a suicidal crisis. Never leave the patient alone, even if he or she no longer threatens harm to himself or herself, as it may be a ploy to facilitate the attempt. You may have to submit yourself to much verbal assault and be required to fulfill seemingly childish or unreasonable acts to buy time with the patient. Never lie to such a patient, as he or she is acutely aware of these responses, and your lying will instill more distrust.

18. (B) When approaching any scene, caution on your part may save your life. Listen for clues as to what is going on inside the house before entering. To avoid being in the path of a shot fired through a door, stand to the side of doors and identify yourself. You may have to wait for the police to secure the scene before care can be initiated.

19. (B) In the case of a suicidal crisis, it is helpful to know if the patient has an actual plan for his death or is just contemplating action. It is also helpful to know if he has tried before. If so, the chances are that he will try again and be successful. Talk openly; using the word "suicide" is

okay since it is his idea. Do not attempt to forcibly gain access, as this may cause injury to yourself or frighten the patient into making good his threat.

20. (D) When approaching and caring for a violent patient, leave yourself an escape route. Only one rescuer should talk. Do not criticize the patient; be professional. You may receive a great deal of verbal abuse. Do not take it personally but remain calm and continue to try to talk the patient down. Always keep the patient's hands in sight.

21. (B) When caring for a paranoid patient, interview family and friends in the presence of the patient. This will let the patient feel less suspicious. Look at the patient, use eye contact, and be sincere, but don't stare. Do not take sides with the patient; remain caring but neutral. Do not lie to this patient, as he or she already distrusts you. Don't reinforce the patient's paranoia.

22. (B) Heroin use causes euphoria, drowsiness, insensitivity to pain, nausea, vomiting, watery eyes, and runny nose. Methamphetamines can increase alertness, talkativeness, loss of appetite, and mood elevation. Cocaine use causes euphoria, restlessness, elevated blood pressure, and heart rate. Marijuana use causes red eyes, dry mouth, reduced concentration, euphoria, and altered perceptions.

23. (C) A PCP patient should be cared for in a dimly lit room, with ears plugged to reduce outside noise. A soft, low voice should be used. Do not attempt to talk the PCP hallucination patient down as in other hallucinogenic drug cases, as it may further aggravate him or her.

24. (C) It is imperative that intoxicated or emotionally disturbed patients be thoroughly examined for medical problems. Always seek out medic alert tags or cards and ask the patient if he or she is on any medication. It is a good practice to always ask if the patient is a diabetic.

25. (D) A patient presenting with signs and symptoms of watery eyes, a runny nose, and slight euphoria could be using a stimulant such as cocaine. The blood pressure, pulse, and respiratory rates are typically elevated in a person using stimulants. The person could have a cold, too! Use of stimulants, legal or illegal, is a police matter, not an EMS concern in this case.

26. (B) When dealing with family members of a deceased patient, it is often helpful if the family is allowed time with the deceased. Allow family members to express feelings; some may cry, while others express anger or denial. If asked directly if the person has died, you should be truthful and express sorrow and caring.

14 Transportation, Patient Handling, and Scene Management

This chapter places heavy emphasis on ambulance operation, including emergency driving skills and aeromedical operations. The topic of secondary patient transfer is also examined. Often, EMTs will be summoned to provide interhospital transfers of acutely ill patients. Without a basic knowledge of proper monitoring and care for these individuals, you can place the patient's life in jeopardy and expose yourself to possible litigation.

Other topics to be reviewed are extrication and communications. These activities are important for the EMT to master because they directly support actual patient care given at the scene and en route to the hospital.

1. What is the recommended minimum following distance between emergency vehicles traveling in an emergency mode?

   A. 100 feet.
   B. 200 feet.
   C. 300 feet.
   D. 500 feet.

2. When operating an ambulance in an emergency mode, you must always:

   A. Pass on the left.
   B. Use the siren.
   C. Exercise due regard.
   D. Display the "Star of Life."

3. What percentage of ambulance responses are true life-and-death situations?

   A. Less than 1%.
   B. Less than 5%.
   C. 10% to 20%.
   D. 20% to 25%.

4. Select the correct statement regarding handling characteristics of a motor vehicle.

   A. When a vehicle accelerates, weight is shifted to the front tires, causing understeering.
   B. When a vehicle accelerates, weight is shifted to the rear tires, causing understeering.
   C. When a vehicle decelerates, weight is shifted forward, causing understeering.
   D. When a vehicle decelerates, weight is shifted to the rear, causing oversteering.

5. During an emergency response, you approach a controlled (traffic light) intersection. Using your emergency signaling devices, when the traffic light turns red for your direction, you should:

   A. Proceed through the intersection without stopping.
   B. Proceed through the intersection, keeping to the far right-hand side.

C. Stop for the traffic light and turn the siren off.
D. Come to a stop and then proceed when the intersection is clear.

6. Safe parking of the ambulance at the scene of a motor vehicle accident should include positioning of the ambulance:

    A. On the left of the cars involved.
    B. On the right of the cars involved.
    C. Just past the cars involved and on their left.
    D. Just past the cars involved and on the curb side of the roadway.

7. During an emergency response, you come up behind a school bus displaying its flashing red lights. You should:

    A. Pass cautiously, using your siren.
    B. Stop and wait until the bus driver signals you on.
    C. Turn your lights and siren off until the bus driver turns his lights off.
    D. Pull into the opposing lanes to pass the bus with a large safety margin.

8. While returning to quarters late one night, you observe an oncoming car approaching you in your lane. Collision seems certain. You should:

    A. Drive to the left.
    B. Drive to the right.
    C. Hold your position.
    D. Sound your siren and flash your lights.

9. The proper following distance for an ambulance traveling 30 mph on dry pavement and good visibility is:

    A. 30 feet.
    B. 40 feet.
    C. 2 seconds.
    D. 3 seconds.

10. Most minor one-vehicle accidents occur while backing. Select the most correct statement.

    A. You (the driver) should open your door and look to the rear when backing.

B. A spotter should be placed to the left rear of the vehicle.
C. The front (steering wheels) tracks in a tighter radius than the rear when backing.
D. A convex (fish-eye) mirror is of great value for backing.

11. Where is the best place to park an ambulance at a suburban residential scene?

    A. Backed into the driveway.
    B. Driven forward into the driveway.
    C. In the street, in front of the driveway.
    D. Halfway into the driveway, with the rear of the ambulance out of the street.

12. Select the most appropriate response with regard to adverse driving conditions.

    A. Emergency signaling devices should be used when driving in heavy fog.
    B. You should watch the center line when approached by oncoming traffic.
    C. The best way to stop on snow or ice is to pump the brakes.
    D. Hydroplaning can occur if the water depth is less than the tire tread depth.

13. Select the correct response with regard to emergency driving.

    A. If the car ahead of you is signaling a left turn, pass on its right side.
    B. You should straddle the center line when driving down a one-way street.
    C. Driving near the center line is preferred when traveling on a two-way street.
    D. You should always use the right lane when turning right on to another street.

14. When parking the ambulance at the scene of an accident that has occurred on a hill, you should:

    A. Park at the base of the hill.
    B. Park at the top of the hill.
    C. Park downwind and downhill.
    D. Park uphill and upwind.

15. Generally, only when a true medical emergency is present should you transport your patient to the hospital using emergency signaling devices. Select the condition that requires the least rapid transportation.

    A. Crushed chest.
    B. Heat stroke.
    C. Bilateral tibia and fibula fractures.
    D. Allergic reactions.

16. From the following choices, select the correct response regarding hazards associated with helicopter operation.

    A. Main rotor blade clearance tends to increase when the blades are turning slowly in windy conditions.
    B. Rotor wash is less severe when you are downwind of the ship.
    C. Patient condition should influence the air medical crew's decision to accept or reject a mission.
    D. Eye contact with the pilot should be established before approaching the aircraft.

17. Which of the following cloud types is most indicative of a potentially hazardous flight condition?

    A. Altostratus.
    B. Cirrus.
    C. Cirrocumulus.
    D. Cumulonimbus.

18. Initial signs or symptoms of hypoxia include:

    A. Depression.
    B. Diminished sight and taste.
    C. Deterioration of visual depth perception.
    D. Excitation, talkativeness.

19. You are assisting a crew in a rotary wing aircraft. As the ship gains altitude, you would expect a normal person's respiratory rate to:

    A. Increase and respiratory depth to increase.
    B. Increase and respiratory depth to decrease.
    C. Decrease and respiratory depth to increase.
    D. Decrease and respiratory depth to decrease.

20. In an unpressurized aircraft, as altitude is increased greatly, several problems can occur including:

    A. Hypoventilation.
    B. Decreased intracranial pressure.
    C. Pneumothorax.
    D. Decreased desire to urinate.

21. Called to an attempted suicide, you find a 30-year-old male who has shot himself in the abdomen and is bleeding profusely. Death appears certain. Just before dying, the patient tells you why he shot himself. You should:

    A. Advise the family of his reasons.
    B. Relay his story to the police.
    C. Relay his story to the medical examiner.
    D. Write the story down on your chart and advise the police.

22. You are called to a small rural hospital to transfer a severely burned female patient to the burn center. The patient has two IVs and cardiac monitoring. As a Basic Life-Support EMT, you should:

    A. Refuse to transport the patient without additional advanced medical personnel.
    B. Transport using red lights and siren.
    C. Transport using just your headlights.
    D. Cover the patient with a moist, sterile burn sheet and transport.

23. You are called upon to transfer an unconscious female patient from one hospital to another. The patient has an endotracheal tube in place. During your transfer, you should:

    A. Suction the tube and mouth with the same catheter.
    B. Listen to both lung fields and pull the tube back slightly if breath sounds are not heard on both sides.
    C. Remove the tube and insert an oral airway.
    D. Position the patient on her side to avoid aspiration.

24. When transporting a patient with a urinary catheter in place, it is important to:

    A. Raise the collection bag above the stretcher.
    B. Keep excess tubing below the level of the collection bag.

C. Keep the collection bag level with the patient.
D. Keep the collection bag below the level of the patient.

25. Mr. Burton is being transferred from one hospital to another. He has an IV in place. Your care for this patient should include:

    A. Observing the infusion site for any swelling or leakage.
    B. Lowering the IV bottle or bag if flow rate decreases.
    C. Turning the IV off if blood is observed in the tubing.
    D. Changing to a 250-mL bag of solution if the flow rate is more than you were directed to maintain.

26. Choose the most appropriate statement regarding MVAs and fires.

    A. Most cars that are involved in a head-on collision catch fire.
    B. There is a higher chance of fire after EMTs arrive on the scene of head-on MVAs than just after impact.
    C. A car fire seldom starts after the arrival of emergency personnel.
    D. The EMT should always disconnect the car battery before turning off the ignition key when extricating patients.

27. When approaching a motor vehicle or other type of accident, you should evaluate the stability of the patient's environment before attempting rescue. You should secure or stabilize a hazard:

    A. After you push on it to see if it will move.
    B. Only after caring for life-threatening injuries.
    C. When the fire department arrives to assist with the rescue.
    D. If it appears to be unstable.

28. Which statement describes a patient who is properly prepared for extrication?

    A. All fractures are permanently splinted.
    B. Legs are temporarily splinted to each other and arms are temporarily splinted to the trunk.
    C. Traction splints have been applied.
    D. A cervical collar has been used to properly immobilize the spine.

29. Select the correct statement regarding the moving and care of patients.

    A. All patients should be placed in the ambulance before splinting is completed.

B. Only patients requiring CPR should be moved before all splinting is completed.
C. Patients should be moved prior to care only if danger is present for the patient or others.
D. Unconscious trauma patients should be pulled from the side by their belt loops.

30. When lifting a loaded stretcher, you should lift with your:

    A. Legs bent and back straight.
    B. Legs straight and back bent.
    C. Arms only to protect your back.
    D. Legs slightly bent and back slightly bent.

31. In order to gain access to a patient trapped in an overturned car, you should:

    A. Cut through the floor.
    B. Open doors or crawl through windows.
    C. Roll the car back over and then open doors.
    D. Use a crane to lift the car off its top.

32. You are called to a residential section for a domestic disturbance injury. You will not have PD backup for at least 10 minutes. You should:

    A. Park the ambulance in front of the scene and approach the house from the side.
    B. Not approach the house until the PD secures the scene.
    C. Stand in front of the front door when knocking so the people inside can quickly identify you as an EMT.
    D. Ask the perpetrator to leave the house before entering.

33. Select the most appropriate statement regarding the use of backboards:

    A. A patient in a PCPD and wearing a rigid cervical collar need not be strapped to a backboard.
    B. A patient strapped to backboard need not be turned on his or her side for proper suctioning.

C. A patient affixed to a short spineboard need not be placed on a long board.
D. A long board is preferable to a short spineboard for rapid extrication.

34. In order to gain access to a patient trapped in a motor vehicle, you should first:

A. Break a side glass window.
B. Try all doors.
C. Cut the door lock away.
D. Remove the windshield.

Answers with Rationale

1. **(D)** While the minimum following distance between emergency vehicles is often given as a linear measurement (500 feet is recommended), the driver of the trailing emergency vehicle must keep in mind that time is the important factor. The emergency driver of the second vehicle must allow time for other drivers to recognize his or her presence and either remain stopped or stop again. Some experts advocate each vehicle using a different siren mode to alert traffic and perhaps, other emergency vehicles' approach from different directions.

2. **(C)** When operating an ambulance in an emergency mode, you must always exercise due regard for the safety of others. Due regard would be to compare the actions "of a reasonably careful person, performing similar duties, under similar conditions, to the acts of the person in question." Was enough notice given to other drivers to (1) recognize your vehicle, (2) make a decision to give you passage, and (3) act upon that decision? A "true emergency" must also exist in order for you to exercise emergency vehicle driving privileges.

3. **(B)** Less than 5% of all ambulance responses are true life-and-death emergencies. Good dispatch, route planning, and efficient driving can reduce many of the risks associated with driving in an emergency mode.

4. **(B)** The coefficient of friction allows only a finite amount of tire traction to prevail. When a vehicle accelerates, weight is shifted to the rear wheels, causing the front tires to have less adhesion to the ground. Understeering can occur. During deceleration the opposite weight shift occurs, and the vehicle rear end may "wash out" and spin.

5. **(D)** It is a good practice to come to a complete stop at any intersection through which you would not normally be allowed to pass. Once all traffic acknowledges your presence (eye contact) and you have their commitment to act (stopped in all directions), you should proceed slowly. Local policy or state statute may prohibit the use of emergency signaling devices, in which case you can proceed only as another vehicle would.

6. **(D)** Generally, the best place to park an ambulance is just beyond the scene, close to the right shoulder. This provides good access and protection to the patient loading zone. You should not impede traffic any more than is necessary. If feasible, park with the ambulance faced in the direction you would take to go to the hospital. Your personal protection, and that of your patient, may determine the need to park a police unit, rescue, or fire apparatus in such a manner as to provide a barrier to approaching traffic.

7. **(B)** When approaching a school bus that is displaying its flashing lights, turn off your siren and stop and wait for the bus driver to signal you to pass. The siren will excite and confuse the children and make the bus driver's task of securing your safe right-of-way more difficult.

8. **(B)** When faced with an almost certain accident, practice defensive driving by choosing an escape route that will be the least destructive to you. Choose the right side of the road in case the other driver sees you and reacts by returning to his side of the roadway. Flashing your lights could actually "blind" a driver temporarily, increasing the risk of collision.

9. **(D)** The proper following distance for a vehicle such as an ambulance is a 3-second margin. Applying the 3-second rule, the ambulance should be able to maintain a safe following distance for dry pavement and good visibility. The 3-second margin is determined by watching the leading vehicle's rear bumper pass a stationary object (sign post, beverage can, etc.) and then counting off the time it takes for your front bumper to pass the object. This margin should be increased when experiencing adverse road surface or vision problems.

10. **(B)** A spotter should be placed to the left rear of the vehicle when reversing. The spotter should use deliberate hand signals. The driver must continue to monitor mirrors at all times. A convex mirror distorts depth perception and should not be relied upon for backing. Since the rear wheels track a much tighter radius than the front, it is important for the driver to constantly monitor the front of the vehicle while backing. This cannot be done if the driver is hanging out the door looking toward the rear. Keep in mind the vehicle pivots at the tires, not the bumpers, so turns should begin as the tires reach the turning point.

11. (C) The best place to park an ambulance at a suburban residential scene is in the street, usually at the foot of the driveway. This position allows easy access while avoiding the need for backing, a very dangerous activity. If a violent situation is at all anticipated, park the vehicle before reaching the scene, well out of any possible line of gunfire.

12. (D) Hydroplaning can occur at higher speeds, even if the depth of the water on the road is less than the depth of the tire tread. Reduce your speed immediately if the vehicle ahead is not leaving tracks on the road. Contrary to popular opinion, the brakes should not be pumped on a slick (rain, ice, snow) road surface. Pumping causes a locking of the wheels and a loss of steering while the tires slide. The brakes should be applied slowly and held at a point just before sliding occurs. If a turn must be made, some brake effort will need to be reduced in order for the tires to develop cornering force. In adverse visibility conditions, the emergency signaling devices should not be operated. Just because your lights and siren are activated, your ability to see is not improved. Never outdrive your visibility. Do not look directly at the headlights of oncoming traffic. Instead, look toward the right side of the road in order to maintain your lane.

13. (C) When responding to an emergency on a two-way street, usually the best place to position your vehicle is crowding the center line. This position accomplishes three things: (1) lets the traffic ahead see you in their left sideview mirrors, (2) telegraphs your intent to pass, and (3) allows the oncoming traffic to see you. Do not pass on the right because the lead driver may try to pull to the curb on the right. Do not turn right from the right-hand lane because your vehicle will be visually shielded from traffic approaching on the cross street. Center street positioning on a one-way street does not allow eye contact with drivers in the left lanes; thus, passing is unsafe.

14. (D) Proper placement of the ambulance at the scene of an accident on a hill is generally uphill from the scene. This will keep you and the vehicle out of danger areas caused by gasoline or chemical spills. Dangerous fumes often collect in low-lying areas. Approach from upwind when possible. Visual warning devices should be placed on both sides of the accident scene to allow time for oncoming traffic to stop safely.

15. (C) Bilateral tibia and fibula fractures are certainly severe injuries. However, they probably will not rapidly lead to death. Crushed chest, heat stroke, and allergic reactions are true emergency cases.

16. (D) Eye contact with the pilot should always be established before approaching the aircraft. The pilot may then give you a hand signal inviting you to approach the ship. All personnel should be alert to the hazards of the tail rotor, especially because it is difficult to see when in operation. Main rotor blades tend to flex downward, especially when turning slowly in windy conditions. The effects of rotor wash are dramatically increased downwind from the aircraft. The degree of patient injury or illness should have absolutely no bearing on the pilot's decision regarding the potential risk of a flight.

17. (D) Vertical development of the cumulonimbus cloud identifies thunderstorm activity, one of the most significant weather patterns relative to flight operations. Thunderstorm activity can include hail, strong vertical currents, and wind shears. Observation of this type of weather pattern near or at the scene of a medical emergency could dictate if aeromedical services should be requested. Altostratus clouds are found at altitudes up to 45,000 feet and do not signify any significant phenomena. Cirrus and cirrocumulus are high altitude, "wispy" clouds, which may indicate the approach of more overcast weather.

18. (D) Initial signs and symptoms of hypoxia that could result from increases in altitude include general hyperactivity, talkativeness, active movements, and excitation. Later stages include depression, impaired reasoning and working ability, and deterioration of visual field/depth perception. Symptoms of continued hypoxia include diminished sensory input and inability to rationalize from sensory input of sight, sound, taste, and pain.

19. (A) As altitude increases, the stimulus to breathe progressively increases causing an increase in both the rate and depth of normal respirations. A severely ill patient's respiratory state may be already compromised because of the disease process, thus requiring supplemental oxygen at higher flow rates than might be needed at ground level.

20. (C) As altitude is increased greatly in an unpressurized aircraft, barometric pressure decreases. This can lead to the development of a

pneumothorax while in flight. Predisposing factors for the development of a pneumothorax include bleb formation, chest injury, asthma, emphysema, and a patient being mechanically ventilated. Increased altitude can result in increased intracranial pressure due to expansion of air in the skull. This could be experienced by a patient with a severe head injury. Patients with basilar skull fractures and mid-face fractures are also predisposed to pneumocephalus. Respiratory rate will increase with increased altitude. At higher altitudes, the urge to void will also increase.

21. (D) When given any statements or directions by a dying patient, always write them down, in the patient's own words, as soon as possible. This information should then be relayed to the police, both in an oral report and in writing.

22. (A) When called to provide secondary transfer of patients from one hospital to another, don't be afraid to refuse transportation without adequate medical assistance. A nurse or paramedic may be needed to properly care for this burn patient should her condition change en route. These professionals may also help you determine the mode of transportation (emergency or nonemergency). Additional dressings and cooling may be detrimental to the patient and increase her body's heat loss.

23. (B) During the transfer of a patient with an endotracheal tube in place, the lungs should be listened to each time the patient is moved to ensure proper placement of the tube. Should you lose breath sounds on one side, slightly adjust the ET tube by pulling it back about one-quarter inch. Do not remove the tube. If you need to suction the tube, do so, but avoid the use of the same catheter for oral suctioning. Avoid prolonged suction.

24. (D) A urinary catheter collection system should be kept below the level of the patient's bladder, avoiding any low spots in the tubing between the catheter and collection bag. This can be accomplished by taping the tubing in a loop to the stretcher.

25. (A) While caring for Mr. Burton, you should observe his IV site for any swelling or leakage. If a large mass develops under the skin, turn the IV off and contact your Medical Control. If the flow decreases in rate, rais-

ing the bag or repositioning his arm may be all that is needed. Do not remove the IV unless directed to do so.

26. (C) Car fires seldom occur after rescue personnel arrive at the scene of an accident. Most fires start at or just after impact. Simply turning off accessories and the ignition reduces much of the electrical fire danger. If a battery is disconnected, it will arc if any current (clock, dome light) is being drawn.

27. (D) You should stabilize the working environment as soon as you suspect that it may be unstable. This can be done by using cribbing or ropes. Even life-threatening injuries may have to wait until it is safe for you to proceed.

28. (B) Temporary splinting of extremities is often all that can be done before extricating a patient to a better working area. Traction splints are very difficult to apply inside a mangled automobile. Cervical collars do little to immobilize the C-spine. The use of backboards and the assistance of several EMTs is recommended for any extrication involving a patient suspected of spinal injuries.

29. (C) Patients should not be moved before proper and complete emergency care is rendered unless patients or rescuers are in dangerous environments. Hazardous environments could include the dangers of fire, hazardous chemicals, toxic fumes, vehicle traffic, or cave-ins. When a patient must be moved prior to proper immobilization, always pull along the long axis of the body, caring for the head and neck.

30. (A) When lifting any heavy object, such as a loaded stretcher, you should keep your back as straight as possible and do the lifting with your more powerful legs. Lift the stretcher by its frame, not the patient side rails.

31. (B) Access to a patient trapped in an overturned car may be gained by crawling through windows or opening doors. Never roll a car back over. The floor would be extremely difficult to cut through. Keep in mind that access is necessary only to allow you to examine and treat a patient. A large opening can later be developed for the extrication phase.

32. (B) It is strongly advised that you not enter a domestic disturbance scene until it is secured by the PD. Park several blocks from the scene until the scene is secured. This is an extremely dangerous situation that requires police intervention prior to your rendering care.

33. (D) A long board may be used rapidly for an extrication from a dangerous environment or for a patient who is rapidly deteriorating. Once the patient is placed on a long board he or she must be securely strapped to the device. This is a frequently overlooked activity. Should the patient's condition deteriorate (e.g., airway problems), the patient will need to be turned to the side and the airway suctioned while the spine is maintained in alignment. Short spineboards are excellent devices for moving a patient from a sitting position to a long board while protecting the spine. Their use is very appropriate if time (most cases) permits their application. Remember, the head and neck are secured only after the trunk has been immobilized.

34. (B) Before making an attempt at forceful entry, always check to see if doors are unlocked or windows open. This is true of houses as well as motor vehicles. Even the best EMT forgets this rule from time to time.

15 Situational Reviews

This final chapter is devoted to the topics of multiple-systems trauma and general patient examination and care. Questions are included on triage, patient assessment, and scene management. Your attention is directed to the proper order of events in the rendering of care. Most of the situations presented are re-creations of actual events.

The objective of this chapter is to help you integrate your cognitive knowledge and applied psycho-motor skills into a consistent, medically-appropriate treatment routine. The chapter should be of considerable benefit to EMTs preparing for the practical skills portion of their certification examination.

During an electrical storm, you are called to a golf course to care for a man who has been struck by lightning. Upon arrival, you discover a male in his early 30s suffering from cardiopulmonary arrest. Your response to the scene took 18 minutes.

1. Your initial action upon arrival at the scene will be to:

    A. Start CPR.
    B. Pronounce the man dead.
    C. Avoid touching the patient, as he may contain electricity.
    D. Call the power company to check the man for voltage.

2. Just after arriving at the golf course, you feel the hair on your head standing up. You should:

    A. Get under a tree.
    B. Jump in the pond next to the green.
    C. Lie flat on the ground.
    D. Continue care, as lightning never strikes twice in the same place.

3. During your care for the golfer struck by lightning, you should:

    A. Hyperextend his neck to ensure an adequate airway.
    B. Examine him for a severe spinal injury.
    C. Use a compression rate of 60 times per minute when performing two-person CPR.
    D. Apply the pneumatic counter-pressure device to combat cardiogenic shock.

4. The most appropriate statement regarding a patient killed by lightning is that:

    A. Severe burns are always present in cases involving lightning deaths.
    B. Death occurs immediately.
    C. Death is usually caused by respiratory arrest.
    D. Death is usually caused by cardiac arrest.

Arriving at the scene of a one-car rollover, you find a young female slumped over behind the wheel of her car. The vehicle shows heavy damage.

5. You should first check the MVA patient for:

    A. Airway and breathing.

B. Severe bleeding.
C. Pulse.
D. Spinal injury.

6. You determine the patient is not breathing and has an easily palpated lump on the back of her neck. Next you should:

    A. Apply traction to her neck.
    B. Apply traction and straighten her neck.
    C. Insert an oral airway.
    D. Open her airway using the jaw thrust maneuver.

7. A crushed steering wheel found in a car accident would lead you to suspect possible injury to a patient's:

    A. Liver.
    B. Appendix.
    C. Lumbar spine.
    D. Pancreas.

8. The woman is having difficulty in breathing, even though you have provided her with an adequate airway. Her chest seems to be working too hard, moving in and out at the same time. You should suspect her respiratory problem is being caused by:

    A. Her neck injury.
    B. A ruptured diaphragm.
    C. A flail chest.
    D. Tension pneumothorax.

9. The woman has been immobilized on a short spineboard. Her respiratory problem is under control. She has bilateral deformity of her knees. Crepitation is heard. You should:

    A. Apply two traction splints.
    B. Splint both legs together.
    C. Apply air splints.
    D. Examine distal pulses.

10. The woman's vital signs indicate that she is going into shock. You are not authorized to apply pneumatic counter-pressure devices. The most important care you can administer to this patient is to:

    A. Apply ice to all fractures to reduce bleeding.

B. Administer high-concentration O₂.
C. Apply warm blankets to preserve body heat.
D. Elevate her feet to at least 18 inches above the level of her heart.

You have been dispatched to a chemical refinery blast. From miles away, you can see heavy, black smoke and flames shooting 300 feet into the sky. The fire department directs you to two men who have been burned. The first patient has second-degree burns on both arms, both legs, and his head. The second patient has first-degree burns on his face, head, and both arms. He is having difficulty in breathing; his nose hairs are singed.

11. How would you rate the burns received by the second patient?

    A. Moderate.
    B. Minor.
    C. Mild.
    D. Critical.

12. What is your immediate care for the first patient?

    A. Cover with burn sheet.
    B. Immerse in cold water.
    C. Wrap legs in sterile aluminum foil.
    D. Apply Vaseline gauze to his facial burns.

You are called to the scene of an unknown illness. Your patient is a 66-year-old female named Rose. She has a history of emphysema. Rose's vital signs are respirations 22, pulse 130, and BP 80/50. Her chief complaint is that she has observed bright-red blood in her stool for several days.

13. The term used for passage of bright-red blood in the stool is:

    A. Hematemesis.
    B. Melena.
    C. Dysphagia.
    D. Hematochezia.

14. Proper care for Rose would include:

    A. Administration of O₂.
    B. Elevation of her head during transportation.

C. Application of ice to her abdomen.
D. Ask Medical Control for advice.

15. Your service is authorized to apply pneumatic counter-pressure devices. How should you use the device on Rose?

    A. Inflate leg compartments only, as the abdomen is probably bleeding.
    B. Inflate all compartments to maximum pressure or 100 mmHg.
    C. Inflate all compartments until her systolic pressure is between 100 and 110 mmHg.
    D. Avoid using device, as it is not indicated.

16. During her transportation to the hospital, Rose suddenly collapses. She is in cardiopulmonary arrest. You should:

    A. Deflate the PCPD and start CPR.
    B. Provide two breaths and palpate the pulse.
    C. Administer a precordial thump.
    D. Not attempt CPR, as she obviously has no blood left to circulate.

You have been called to the scene of a gas station holdup. You find the attendant unconscious in the office. He has been stabbed several times. A knife is impaled in his left thigh and his shirt is blood-soaked around the area of his left clavicle.

17. After checking the attendant's airway, your next action should be to:

    A. Apply pressure to the thigh wound.
    B. Expose the chest.
    C. Take vital signs.
    D. Check for a femur fracture.

18. Your partner has applied direct pressure to the patient's thigh wound after you have exposed the chest. Vital signs are pulse 130, resp. 22, BP 100/60. A sucking chest wound is present. Your next action should be to:

    A. Administer O_2.
    B. Elevate the legs.
    C. Seal the chest wound.
    D. Remove the knife for evidence.

19. The attendant is experiencing dyspnea and hemoptysis. You should suspect:

    A. Subcutaneous emphysema.
    B. Hemothorax.
    C. Myocardial contusion.
    D. Pericardial tamponade.

20. The police on the scene have requested you to preserve the evidence. You should:

    A. Carefully remove the knife.
    B. Immobilize the knife.
    C. Cut the clothing off by starting at the hole created by the knife.
    D. Suggest photographing the knife.

21. You have sealed the sucking chest wound and dressed the thigh. Next, you should:

    A. Take a new set of vital signs.
    B. Administer O_2.
    C. Elevate the legs.
    D. Transport the patient on his injured side.

22. Within five minutes of your initial treatment, the condition of the attendant worsens. Respirations become more labored, the pulse weakens, and neck veins become engorged. You should suspect:

    A. Hemorrhagic shock from the thigh wound.
    B. Tension pneumothorax.
    C. Hemoptysis.
    D. Paradoxical thorax.

23. The recommended treatment for the condition in Question 22 is:

    A. Elevating the legs to 18 inches.
    B. Occasionally releasing the chest dressing.
    C. Slightly raising the patient's head.
    D. Immobilizing the injured chest wall.

24. Upon your arrival at the Emergency Department, your prime concern is to:

    A. Report initial vital signs.

B. Preserve the evidence.
  C. Accurately complete your run report.
  D. Report changes in the patient's condition while en route.

You are working with a private ambulance service. You receive a call to respond to a switchyard for men down. You are advised that a rail tank car is leaking chlorine gas.

25. How would you handle this response?

    A. Not respond, as this is a fire department responsibility.
    B. Approach the scene from upwind.
    C. Approach the scene from downwind.
    D. Approach using the portable O_2 to protect yourself.

26. As you approach the switchyard, you observe a gaseous cloud. What color cloud would you expect from chlorine gas?

    A. Red.
    B. Yellow.
    C. Blue.
    D. Green.

27. The fire department has secured the chlorine gas leak and carried two men to a safe area for treatment. You should:

    A. Irrigate them with ammonia.
    B. Irrigate them with water.
    C. Administer O_2 and irrigate them with water.
    D. Transport them with the patient compartment heaters on full force.

28. The two men rescued from the chlorine gas leak will most likely have severe:

    A. Burns.
    B. Respiratory distress.
    C. Cherry-red skin color.
    D. Frostbite.

You have responded to the home of a woman in labor. During your exam of the woman for crowning, a sudden gush of fluid erupts from her vagina. The umbilical cord is about 2 inches outside of the vagina.

29. Your first action in providing care will be to:

    A. Cut the cord.
    B. Wrap the cord in dry, sterile dressings.
    C. Push the cord back into the vagina.
    D. Raise the woman's hips and administer high-concentration O_2.

30. During a normal delivery, when would you suction a newborn?

    A. Suction immediately after the head is delivered.
    B. Suction after the head and shoulders are delivered.
    C. Suction only after the entire body is delivered.
    D. Suction one minute after the entire body is delivered if infant is not yet breathing on his or her own.

31. After the delivery of the infant, you should transport:

    A. Immediately.
    B. As soon as the placenta is delivered.
    C. In five minutes if the placenta is not delivered.
    D. After the police have arrived to pronounce the baby alive.

32. The newborn infant has a very soft head, smells bad, and appears lifeless. He is not breathing and has no pulse. You should:

    A. Give four breaths and then start compression at 60 times per minute.
    B. Give two breaths and compress at 80 times per minute.
    C. Give two breaths and compress the infant's sternum using a 5:1 ratio.
    D. Not start CPR.

33. The mother is bleeding heavily from her vagina just after the delivery of the placenta. You should:

    A. Pack the vagina with sterile dressings.
    B. Massage the uterus and place a sterile pad over the vagina.

C. Apply pneumatic counter-pressure devices but do not inflate the abdomen.
D. Elevate the patient's head, administer high-level O_2, and place her legs together.

34. Immediately after giving birth, the mother experiences shortness of breath, increased heart rate, and low blood pressure. You should suspect:

    A. Psychogenic shock.
    B. Air embolism.
    C. Abruptio placenta.
    D. Placenta previa.

You are dispatched to a downtown area. There is a report of a sniper firing shots. One elderly man is known to be shot and is still lying in the middle of the street.

35. Your response to the scene should:

    A. Be handled in the emergency mode, watching for police units also converging on the scene.
    B. Be handled without red light or siren so as not to alert the sniper of your arrival.
    C. Not be made until the sniper is in custody.
    D. Include approaching the rear of the address without lights or siren, wearing a red cross and waving a white flag.

36. The police are able to remove the elderly man from the street and drag him to a safety zone. The man has been shot in the abdomen. Your first action is to:

    A. Open the patient's airway.
    B. Remove all clothing from around the wound.
    C. Examine for an exit wound.
    D. Apply direct pressure to the abdomen.

37. The gunshot victim has a pulse of 140, resp. 30, and BP of 80/40. His airway is open. There is an exit wound in the middle of the lower back. Bone chips are visible. You should first:

    A. Pack both wounds with dry, sterile dressings.

B. Apply moist dressings to any evisceration and dry dressings to the back wound.
C. Apply a cervical collar.
D. Apply rotating tourniquets and elevate the feet.

38. This patient is best treated by use of:

    A. Ice to reduce bleeding and swelling.
    B. Long spineboard, as the back wound indicates spinal involvement.
    C. Pneumatic counter-pressure device.
    D. Occlusive dressings and sterile aluminum foil.

39. The best position in which to transport this patient is on his:

    A. Left side.
    B. Back, with feet elevated 8 to 12 inches.
    C. Stomach, in a level position.
    D. Back, with head elevated slightly and turned to the side.

40. Should it become necessary to apply a pneumatic counter-pressure device to this patient, you should consider his evisceration and:

    A. Inflate only the leg compartments.
    B. Inflate the device to maximum as soon as possible.
    C. First apply a short spineboard and then inflate until the patient's systolic pressure reaches 120 mmHg.
    D. Inflate leg units first, then abdominal until the patient's systolic BP reaches 100–110 mmHg.

41. During the transfer of the patient to the Emergency Department, he begins to vomit. You should:

    A. Hyperextend his neck to ensure a patent airway.
    B. Apply suction for periods of less than 10 seconds to clear the airway.
    C. Avoid turning the patient on his side and further complicating the spinal injury.
    D. Insert an oral airway to facilitate suctioning.

You are dispatched to a small apartment complex about five minutes from your quarters. A frantic mother explains that her 6-year-old daughter,

Becky, has mistakenly ingested dishwashing liquid she thought was lemon juice.

42. You will care for Becky by:

    A. Diluting the soap with milk or water.
    B. Avoiding the use of water, as it may cause suds in the stomach.
    C. Immediately inducing vomiting.
    D. Neutralizing the dish soap with soda water.

43. Becky will most likely exhibit signs of:

    A. Nausea and diarrhea.
    B. Rapid loss of consciousness.
    C. Severe burns about the lips and mouth.
    D. Shock, including pale skin, rapid pulse and respirations.

You have been called to a men's correctional institution to care for a number of injured inmates. A small riot flared up and tear gas has been used.

44. While triaging the patients, you know which one of the following will require the first care?

    A. Teary-eyed patient with respiratory wheeze, broken lower left arm.
    B. Unconscious patient with stab wound in the abdomen and heavy blood loss.
    C. Patient with shotgun wound to the head, with brain tissue visible, irregular gasping respirations, and dilated pupils.
    D. Conscious, combative patient with shotgun wound to the left shoulder.

45. Your initial care for the inmate with the shotgun wound to the head should include:

    A. Applying pressure dressings to control bleeding.
    B. Placing him in a feet-elevated shock position.
    C. Inserting an oral airway and administering O_2.
    D. Applying pneumatic counter-pressure device.

46. Proper care for the inmate with the stab wound in his abdomen includes:

    A. Applying a pneumatic counter-pressure device (authorized equipment for your service).
    B. Raising the patient's legs by the use of pillows to promote blood return.
    C. Placing the patient on his side to promote an adequate airway.
    D. Administering O_2 at 4 liters and applying ice packs to reduce bleeding.

47. In addition to controlling the bleeding of the inmate's (Patient D) shoulder wound, your priority should be:

    A. Check for distal neurovascular status.
    B. Administer O_2 to combat the effects of the tear gas.
    C. Insert an oral airway to quiet the inmate.
    D. Suspect his combativeness is a result of the lifestyle that led to his incarceration.

48. After the answer to Question 47, the next priority for the patient with a shotgun wound in the shoulder should be to:

    A. Check for distal neurovascular status.
    B. Administer O_2 to combat the effects of the tear gas.
    C. Insert an oral airway to quiet the inmate.
    D. Suspect his combativeness is a result of the lifestyle that led to his incarceration.

49. Your first priority in treating the inmate with teary eyes, respiratory wheeze, and a fractured lower arm should be to:

    A. Administer O_2.
    B. Irrigate the eyes with a neutralizing agent.
    C. Immobilize the arm with an air splint.
    D. Check and record vital signs.

50. The inmate with the stab wound in the abdomen is dark-skinned. The best place to check for adequate oxygenation is in his:

    A. Mouth.
    B. Axilla (armpit).
    C. Ear lobe.
    D. Feet.

51. During an examination of a conscious male trauma patient, your first action in examining him for spinal injury should be to ask the patient:

    A. To say whether or not he can feel your touch.
    B. To grasp your hands.
    C. To try to move his back.
    D. To say whether or not he has any neck or back pain.

52. The second action during the exam of a patient with a possible spinal injury should be to ask the patient:

    A. To say whether or not he can feel your touch.
    B. To grasp your hands.
    C. To try to move his back.
    D. To say whether or not he has any back pain.

53. You are dispatched to a street corner location for a patient experiencing seizures. Upon your arrival, you should:

    A. Administer 2 L/min oxygen via nasal cannula.
    B. Protect the patient by restraining his arms and legs.
    C. Place a tongue blade between the patient's front teeth.
    D. Protect the patient's head by placing pillows around him.

54. The seizure has been continuous for nearly 12 minutes. You should:

    A. Transport immediately.
    B. Administer Dilantin.
    C. Administer sugar cubes.
    D. Apply ice packs to the patient's head.

Search and Rescue team members have just located a 4-year-old diabetic boy who has been lost for two days in rugged terrain. It is late fall, and the nights have been cold and damp. The child is unconscious.

55. You would not expect the child's unconsciousness to be caused by:

    A. Hypothermia.
    B. Exhaustion.
    C. Diabetic coma.
    D. Insulin shock.

56. This child will most likely have:

    A. Kussmaul respirations.
    B. Normal pulse.
    C. Normal breath odor.
    D. Drooling.

57. Your care for this child should include:

    A. Administration of sugar cubes.
    B. Immersion in hot water of 105°F to 110°F.
    C. Hyperventilation by bag-valve-mask device with 100% O_2.
    D. Covering with warm blankets.

You are called to the scene of a farming accident, and find a 42-year-old male (Spike) who has had his left hand cut off by a cornpicker. He has a pulse of 130, rapid respirations (24), and BP of 100/60.

58. To control Spike's bleeding, you should:

    A. Apply a tourniquet to his forearm.
    B. Apply a tourniquet to his upper arm.
    C. Elevate his arm and apply direct pressure to the stump.
    D. Wrap the stump in aluminum foil and elevate.

59. Proper care for the amputated hand includes:

    A. Immersing it in a bucket of ice.
    B. Covering it with aluminum foil.
    C. Placing it on Spike's chest to preserve body heat.
    D. Wrapping it in a sterile dressing and placing it in a cool container.

60. You have controlled Spike's bleeding. What would be the best position in which to transport him?

    A. Supine, with feet elevated and left arm elevated.
    B. Semi-sitting, with arm elevated.
    C. Semi-sitting, with arms level.
    D. Supine, with PCPD inflated.

61. If Spike begins to show signs of shock, you should expect his:

    A. BP to rise and pulse rate to fall.
    B. BP to rise slightly, then fall as the pulse rate increases.

C. BP to fall, pulse rate to slowly drop off, and respirations to slow.
D. BP to fall, pulse rate to fall, and respiration rate to rise.

62. Called to the scene of a patient having difficulty breathing, you find a slender male patient smoking a cigarette and leaning forward in a chair with his hands on his knees using his accessory muscles for respiration. These classical signs are of a patient suffering from:

    A. Hyperventilation syndrome.
    B. Asthma.
    C. Pulmonary edema.
    D. Emphysema.

63. Proper care for the patient in Question 62 includes:

    A. Transporting in a sitting position.
    B. Administering high-concentration O_2.
    C. Encouraging the patient to take shallow breaths.
    D. Transporting in a feet-up position.

The police dispatcher has requested an ambulance. He is unsure of the situation but believes an officer has been shot while trying to apprehend a male suspected of being on a "drug trip." You arrive and discover the officer has been shot in the back. He is wearing a bullet-proof vest. The officer has no open wounds but has swelling and ecchymosis on his back directly over the thoracic spine.

64. You determine that pain during motion is present. You have applied ice to the officer's back. You should then:

    A. Apply a long spineboard and C-collar.
    B. Apply a sling and swathe.
    C. Elevate the officer's feet.
    D. Administer O_2.

65. Other officers have apprehended the assailant. He is demonstrating bizarre behavior and is unable to speak. The assailant's eyes are involuntarily moving about in both horizontal and vertical planes. You should suspect:

    A. Head injury.
    B. PCP ingestion.

C. Barbiturate overdose.
D. Marijuana intoxication.

66. When dealing with the assailant, you should:

    A. "Talk him down."
    B. Check him for injuries.
    C. Place him in a well-lit area.
    D. Shout at the assailant because his hearing is impaired.

67. You should expect this assailant patient to demonstrate signs of:

    A. Increased urine output.
    B. Acute muscle rigidity.
    C. Increased respiratory rate.
    D. Dry skin.

You are called to a nearby cafe. Twenty-year-old Barry is coughing and grasping his throat.

68. Your first action for Barry, who is standing, is to:

    A. Hyperextend his neck.
    B. Encourage him to continue coughing.
    C. Give abdominal thrusts.
    D. Give back blows.

69. After your initial action in Question 68, Barry falls to the ground, unconscious. You should now:

    A. Hyperextend his neck.
    B. Begin artificial respiration.
    C. Perform abdominal thrusts.
    D. Perform a finger sweep.

70. After your action in Question 69, you should now:

    A. Hyperextend his neck.
    B. Perform abdominal thrusts.
    C. Perform a finger sweep.
    D. Attempt artificial ventilation.

You are called to the scene of a motorcycle accident. The motorcyclist, Larry, was attempting to pass a car when it suddenly turned left. The cyclist is found unconscious, lying on his stomach in the middle of the street. He is wearing a helmet. He is cyanotic and has an obvious open fracture of his left femur.

71. Your first action of care for Larry should be to:

    A. Remove his helmet.
    B. Apply traction to the neck.
    C. Apply traction to the fractured femur.
    D. Open the airway.

72. Your next action should be to:

    A. Remove his helmet.
    B. Apply traction to the neck.
    C. Apply traction to the fractured femur.
    D. Open the airway.

73. You should now care for Larry by:

    A. Administering O_2.
    B. Applying a cervical collar.
    C. Recording vital signs.
    D. Applying a traction splint.

Larry is now receiving O_2, his airway is open, your partner is maintaining neck traction, and vitals are pulse 140, resp. 26 and shallow, BP 70/44. Larry has one dilated pupil. The helmet has been removed to better access his airway.

74. You should now apply a:

    A. Long spineboard.
    B. Traction splint.
    C. PCPD.
    D. Cervical collar.

75. After your action in Question 74, you should apply a:

    A. Long spineboard.

B. Traction splint.
C. PCPD.
D. Cervical collar.

Larry is now on a long spineboard, has a PCPD inflated to 100 mmHg, and has a traction splint applied to the outside of the PCPD. He suddenly stops breathing.

76. You should first check Larry's:

    A. Pulse.
    B. Airway.
    C. Blood pressure.
    D. Pupils.

77. You determine Larry is in full cardiopulmonary arrest. You are alone in the back of the ambulance. You should:

    A. Start CPR with five compressions as his airway is already open.
    B. Start CPR with two breaths.
    C. Check his pulse.
    D. Administer a precordial thump.

You are called to a home where you find Mary Ann, a 27-year-old female, unconscious, cyanotic, with no palpable pulse or respirations. You observe several pill bottles strewn about and a suicide note.

78. Your initial action at the scene will be to:

    A. Open her airway and ventilate.
    B. Notify the police.
    C. Call for the medical examiner.
    D. Avoid mouth-to-mouth resuscitation as you may become contaminated from toxins.

79. If your action was to perform CPR on Mary Ann, you should:

    A. Discontinue CPR after 3 minutes if her color does not improve.
    B. Interrupt the CPR for 45 seconds while you place her in the ambulance.

C. Discontinue CPR if her pupils do not constrict after 3 minutes of CPR.
D. Continue CPR for a long period of time since she may survive due to depression of bodily functions.

80. What is the most appropriate disposition of a suicide note?

    A. Leave it at the scene.
    B. Wait for the police to arrive and then give it to them.
    C. Take it with you to the Emergency Department.
    D. Mail it to the medical examiner if the patient dies.

You are called to a rural road by sheriff's deputies to assist a man trapped in a car. The car has hit a snow bank, the gas tank is empty, and the ignition is on. After breaking the side glass and removing the man, you discover he is red-faced, cool to touch, and unconscious. The odor of alcohol is present.

81. You would most likely expect the patient to be suffering from:

    A. Carbon monoxide poisoning.
    B. Alcohol intoxication.
    C. Hypothermia.
    D. All of the above.

82. What is the probable cause of this accident?

    A. Heart attack.
    B. Carbon monoxide poisoning.
    C. Alcohol intoxication.
    D. Hypothermia.

83. After you observe that the patient has an open airway, you determine he is breathing and has a pulse. You should immediately:

    A. Administer O_2.
    B. Apply warm packs to his extremities.
    C. Record vital signs.
    D. Prepare him for transportation.

You are called to a scene where a 6-year-old girl, Dawn, has fallen off her bicycle. A witness explains that she just fell over. She has an obvious deformity of her left elbow. She is limp and sleepy. She is wearing a medic alert bracelet stating she is an epileptic.

84. After opening Dawn's airway, you should:

    A. Administer sugar cubes.
    B. Administer O_2.
    C. Apply neck traction.
    D. Check distal pulses.

85. You have determined that Dawn does not have any injuries other than possibly a dislocated elbow. She does not have a distal pulse in her left arm. It will be nearly a 30-minute transport to the hospital. You should:

    A. Apply gentle in-line traction to straighten the elbow and restore the pulse.
    B. Splint the elbow in place using board splints.
    C. Splint the elbow in the most comfortable position for the patient.
    D. Apply an air splint, as it will return the proper angle to the elbow.

86. The normal respiratory rate for a 6-year-old child is:

    A. 30–40.
    B. 20–30.
    C. 20–25.
    D. 14–26.

87. You are called to the home of a terminally ill man. His wife explains that the man just wants to die at home. You should:

    A. Initiate CPR if arrest occurs.
    B. Isolate the family.
    C. Transport him immediately to the hospital.
    D. Assess whether the family is prepared.

88. A 72-year-old male has no feeling on one side, is drooling from his mouth, and has a BP of 210/140. You should suspect:

    A. Heat stroke.
    B. CVA.

C. Acute MI.
D. Diabetic coma.

89. Which of the following actions would be most appropriate for the patient in Question 88?

    A. Transport on his back with head slightly elevated.
    B. Administer nitroglycerin.
    C. Provide positive-pressure ventilations if his respiratory rate is below 18 times per minute.
    D. Transport on his affected side.

90. You are called to an apparent one-car accident. You arrive at the scene and note that the car has no apparent damage although it is off the shoulder. The unconscious driver, a male in his late 50s, appears cyanotic and diaphoretic. There are no signs of trauma. You should suspect:

    A. Heart attack.
    B. Neurogenic shock.
    C. Head injury.
    D. Seizure.

Answers with Rationale

1. **(A)** CPR should be started on patients who have suffered severe electrical shocks (as from lightning) even after long periods of time. These patients seem to fall outside of the 6-to-10-minute brain death rule. The golfer will not contain any electricity.

2. **(C)** Should you feel the hair on your head start to stand up during an electrical storm, immediately lie down on the ground and keep all of your body (including your head) flat. Avoid trees, as they may attract lightning; stay out of water, as water is an excellent conductor of electricity. Your vehicle may give some protection, as the tires offer insulation. Avoid touching any metal.

3. **(B)** A person who has been struck by lightning often suffers a severe injury to the spine. Do not hyperextend the neck during a resuscitation of this type of patient.

4. **(D)** Lightning need not directly hit someone to cause death. Death is usually a result of a cardiac arrhythmia or arrest. Burns may or may not be present.

5. **(A)** Your initial observation of the patient should be for breathing and airway. You should suspect spinal injury and protect her by using a modified jaw thrust/chin lift maneuver to open the airway.

6. **(D)** With the observance of a neck injury, you should use the jaw thrust maneuver to open her airway. Her neck should not be moved.

7. **(A)** A crushed steering wheel could indicate possible injuries to a patient's liver, spleen, ribs, or lungs.

8. **(C)** You should suspect a flail chest as the cause of her breathing difficulties. The paradoxical movement is your most important clue. Splint or immobilize the flail segment immediately with a sandbag or bulky dressing. Positive-pressure breathing may be required to adequately ventilate this woman.

9. (D) The woman has apparent fractures of both knees. Determine distal neurovascular status in both legs before proceeding with splinting. Avoid traction splints. Do not splint both legs together, as neither is stable. Rigid splints are preferred to air splints for knee injuries.

10. (B) Although often overlooked, administration of high-concentration O_2 is indicated in all patients exhibiting signs of shock. The foot end of the spineboard should be elevated, but not over 12 inches, as any more height increases breathing difficulties.

11. (D) Both burn patients would be classified as having critical burns. Patient 2 has respiratory problems, which place him in the high-priority group.

12. (A) The first patient has 63% of body surface burned. You should cover him with a burn sheet, administer O_2, and treat for shock. Immersion for such a large body surface area is contraindicated, as it may rapidly lead to hypothermia. Aluminum foil should not be used, as it may actually increase the burn by retaining heat.

13. (D) Hematochezia is the term used to describe bright-red blood in the stool. Melena is dark, tarry blood in the stool. Dysphagia is difficulty in swallowing. Hematemesis refers to vomiting of blood.

14. (A) Rose is demonstrating signs of shock and should be treated for it by administering O_2, elevating the lower extremities, and keeping her warm. Do not administer anything to drink.

15. (C) Proper application of the PCPD to Rose would call for all three compartments to be used. Inflation of the abdominal compartment may reduce her internal bleeding. The device should be inflated only enough to raise her systolic BP to between 100 and 110 mmHg.

16. (B) Rose has gone into cardiopulmonary arrest. Open her airway, give two ventilations, 1½–2 seconds each, and palpate the pulse. If the pulse is absent, begin CPR. Do not deflate the PCPD, as this would increase the pooling of blood. A precordial thump is only indicated in monitored situations. Do not perform the thump, as this is no longer considered a BLS procedure.

17. (B) The chest of the gas station attendant must be exposed and rapidly examined for penetrating wounds. A sucking chest wound should be considered as important as an obstructed airway, since it causes a severe compromise to respirations.

18. (C) The sucking chest wound must be sealed to prevent further air from entering the chest cavity and causing a collapsed lung and hypoxia. The seal on the chest wound should be completed just before the patient inhales.

19. (B) Since the attendant is experiencing labored breathing and coughing up blood, you should expect lung injury with bleeding, or hemothorax.

20. (B) The knife should not be removed but should be immobilized in place. Increased tissue, nerve, or vessel damage may occur if the knife is removed. Removal of clothing by cutting through the stab wound area may also destroy evidence.

21. (B) Oxygen should be administered as soon as possible since the respiratory system has suffered a major insult. Everything should be done to reduce hypoxia and increase perfusion. The legs can be elevated after the O_2 is started. The patient may also be transported on his side, injured lung dependent or down. This will reduce the chance of fluids entering the uninjured lung.

22. (B) Increased dyspnea, weaker pulse, and engorged neck veins indicate the development of a tension pneumothorax.

23. (B) When tension pneumothorax is suspected after sealing a chest wound, simply opening the occlusive dressing occasionally during exhalation may allow the excess air to leak and reduce the tension. Air will be heard escaping, and the patient will improve rapidly.

24. (D) The change of status of the patient is of prime importance to the Emergency Department staff. Your timely care for the tension pneumothorax is paramount. Accurate prehospital report forms and continued safeguarding of all the evidence, including clothing, will be important later on. The patient's health is your prime concern.

25. (B) You should approach the switchyard from upwind. Seek out the fire command post and be ready to evacuate. Your portable O_2 will only partially protect your lungs. Full turnouts and air packs are required for this environment.

26. (D) A chlorine gas cloud will be greenish in color.

27. (C) The two men exposed to the chlorine gas will need respiratory support. High-concentration O_2 is indicated. They should also be thoroughly irrigated with water. Start irrigation as soon as the airway and breathing are cared for. Remove patients' clothing during irrigation process.

28. (B) The two men will most likely be in respiratory distress. The skin will be irritated by the chlorine as well.

29. (D) Upon discovering a prolapsed cord, you should raise the woman's hips or place her in a knee-chest position and administer high-concentration O_2. Observe the cord for pulsations and wrap the cord in moist, sterile dressings. Do not attempt to replace the cord. If the infant is crowning, gently push the head up to prevent pressure on the cord.

30. (A) You should suction an infant as soon as the head is delivered. First suction out the mouth and throat, then suction the nose. A newborn is primarily a nose breather. Stimulating the breathing response prior to clearing the mouth and nose may cause the infant to aspirate. The infant should start breathing on his or her own after the mouth and nose are cleared.

31. (B) Unless the mother or infant is in distress, you should allow the placenta to deliver before transporting. Should the placenta not deliver within 20 minutes of the baby, transport at that time. Massage the uterus after the placenta is delivered.

32. (D) A lifeless infant with a very soft head, bad odor, and perhaps blisters on the skin is a stillborn. Do not attempt resuscitation. If in doubt, it is always best to start CPR, giving two breaths and then a 5:1 ratio of compressions at a rate of at least 100 per minute.

33. (B) Gentle massage of the uterus will help the uterus to contract and should reduce bleeding. Cover the vaginal opening with sterile pads.

The PCPD may be indicated if shock occurs. Contact your Medical Control. Always administer high-concentration O_2 to patients who are severely hemorrhaging.

34. (B) A sudden shortness of breath, increase in heart rate, and decrease in blood pressure just after delivery may indicate an air embolism. The mother should be placed on her left side and have O_2 administered. Psychogenic shock (fainting) is not likely to cause shortness of breath. Abruptio placenta and placenta previa occur before the baby is delivered.

35. (A) You would respond to this scene in an emergency mode, unless directed otherwise, being watchful for other emergency vehicles at any intersection. The sniper is certainly aware that he will receive much attention. You should ask the police command post where they would like your unit placed. Do not attempt to approach the sniper, as this is a police matter. The police should keep you in a safe location.

36. (A) Your first patient care action will always be to open and maintain the airway.

37. (B) The gunshot wounds should be dressed with sterile dressings. If bowels are visible, moist dressings sealed with aluminum foil to retain body heat and moisture are indicated. Do not pack the abdominal wound if any evisceration is observed. The bone fragments may be parts of the spine.

38. (C) Application and inflation of a pneumatic counter-pressure device would be the treatment of choice. The patient is exhibiting the signs of shock. The spine should be protected but is secondary to the ensuing shock. Moist dressings sealed with foil are also indicated if bowels protrude outside of the peroneal cavity.

39. (B) This patient should be transported in a supine position, on a long spineboard with the foot end elevated 8 to 12 inches. Airway problems and vomiting should be anticipated.

40. (A) Inflation of the PCPD should be done using only the leg compartments. The pressure should be only that which is required to raise the patient's systolic BP to between 100 and 110 mmHg. Overinflation may actually increase bleeding.

41. (B) If this patient vomits, you must protect his airway by performing oral suctioning. The airway should not be suctioned for periods longer than 10 seconds, as this removes the oxygen available for breathing. If you are unable to manage the airway in this manner, turn the patient. He should be secured to a long spineboard. Keep in mind that the spinal injury is secondary to the airway and life itself.

42. (A) Dilute ingested liquid dish soaps with water or milk. If a large quantity has been ingested, spontaneous vomiting may occur. There is no need to induce vomiting, as there are no corrosive or toxic effects caused by household strength liquid soap.

43. (A) The young girl will most likely develop nausea and diarrhea from the ingestion of the dish soap. The effects of ingesting powder-type detergents used in dishwashers are altogether different. Contact your Medical Control or poison control center for instructions.

44. (B) Although each of the inmates needs immediate care, Patient B is the choice for first care. He is unconscious, so an airway problem is likely, and is bleeding heavily. He is salvageable. Patient A, the second priority for care, has respiratory problems that require O_2 and possible assistance. Patient D is the third priority for care. Patient C is probably mortally wounded; his recovery is unlikely.

45. (C) Initial care for this inmate would be to ensure an adequate airway and administer high-concentration O_2. His respirations should be assisted by bag-valve-mask. The head wound can be loosely dressed. Treatment for shock may do little to save this patient.

46. (A) Should your ambulance service be authorized to use pneumatic counter-pressure devices, your Medical Control will probably instruct you to immediately apply the PCPD. High-concentration O_2 is indicated at 8–10 liters per minute by mask. The patient should be kept in a supine position and only have his legs elevated when on a long spineboard.

47. (B) The inmate with the shoulder wound should have O_2 administered to combat the effects of the tear gas and ensuing shock.

48. (A) After the administration of O_2, the patient's distal neurovascular status should be observed. Then his shoulder should be splinted. Never

insert an airway in a conscious patient. His combativeness may be caused by the shoulder wound's blood loss.

49. (A) The inmate exhibiting respiratory wheeze should immediately have O_2 administered. The vital signs should then be recorded. Irrigate the patient's eyes with water only. Finally, splint the lower arm fracture, immobilizing both the wrist and elbow. Check distal neurovascular status before and after splinting.

50. (A) Dark-skinned patients can be observed for cyanosis or other changes in skin color in the mouth and nail beds.

51. (D) The first part of an examination of a conscious patient suspected of having a spinal injury should be to ask the patient if he or she has any neck or back pain, tingling, or numbness.

52. (A) The second part of the examination should be to check to see if the patient can feel your touch. You can also introduce a pain stimuli, such as a pin prick or pinch. If any finding confirms a spinal injury, instruct the patient not to move, and proceed with immobilization.

53. (D) Use pillows and blankets, especially around the head, to protect the seizure patient from injury. You should not restrain the patient, as this action may further aggravate the problem. Avoid placing anything between the teeth.

54. (A) This patient is considered to be in status epilepticus because the seizure has lasted more than 10 minutes. Transport immediately, as this is a true medical emergency.

55. (D) The 4-year-old diabetic boy has been without insulin for two days. He may have been eating wild foods. Most likely, he will be in a diabetic coma. Hypothermia and exhaustion may also be present.

56. (A) The diabetic coma patient will most likely have Kussmaul respirations as the body attempts to return to a normal pH level. The pulse rate may be elevated, and the blood pressure may be normal or slightly low. Both the pulse rate and BP may be down if hypothermia is present. Drooling and normal breath odor are also associated with insulin shock.

57. (D) Cover the patient with warm blankets and avoid rough handling. Since the child is unconscious, sugar should not be administered orally.

Hyperventilation may actually cause ventricular fibrillation in a hypothermia patient.

58. (C) Control of bleeding from an amputated limb such as Spike's can be accomplished by applying direct pressure to the stump and elevating it above the level of the heart. Many dressings may be required. If this is unsuccessful, locate the pressure point (brachial artery) and apply pressure. Should a tourniquet be needed, apply it just above the elbow.

59. (D) The amputated hand should be wrapped in sterile dressings, placed in a plastic bag, and kept in a cool container. Avoid freezing the hand.

60. (A) Spike would probably be best transported on his back, with legs elevated to prevent shock. The left arm is elevated to reduce bleeding and swelling. The arm should be splinted. The inflation of a PCPD is not yet indicated, as his systolic pressure is above 90 mmHg.

61. (B) Spike's blood pressure may rise slightly as the body vasoconstricts to shunt blood to the vital organs. It will then fall. The pulse rate will increase in an attempt to adequately perfuse the tissue. The respiratory rate may also rise.

62. (D) The slender, smoking patient with dyspnea who leans forward while sitting most likely suffers from emphysema.

63. (A) This patient will be most comfortable if transported in a sitting position. Low-level O_2 (no more than 2 L/min) can be administered to aid the patient. High-level O_2 can depress the hypoxic drive and cause respiratory arrest. The patient should be encouraged to take slow, deep breaths.

64. (A) The officer should be immobilized to protect his thoracic spine. This is best accomplished by application of a long spineboard. Be sure to totally immobilize the spine, monitor vital signs for any changes, and be prepared to clear the airway if necessary.

65. (B) Bizarre behavior, inability to speak, and involuntary eye movement in a vertical plane are all symptoms of Phencyclidine (PCP) ingestion.

66. (B) The PCP "trip" patient may be injured and not realize it, as PCP is an anesthetic. A careful exam is indicated. The PCP patient cannot be talked down as can patients with intoxication from other hallucinogens. He should be kept in a darkened, quiet room or space. Shouting will only aggravate the patient, as hearing becomes more acute while under the influence of PCP.

67. (B) Acute muscle rigidity is often seen in PCP patients. Urine output may decrease. The respiratory rate may slow or cease completely. The skin will probably be moist.

68. (B) Barry is coughing, thus he is moving air. He should be encouraged to continue his coughing.

69. (D) Barry, who is now unconscious with a complete airway occlusion, should have his mouth opened with a tongue-jaw lift and a deep finger sweep performed to remove the foreign body.

70. (D) After clearing foreign material from Barry's airway, you should reposition his head and chin and attempt rescue breathing. If unsuccessful, perform abdominal thrusts to relieve any remaining obstruction.

71. (D) Your first action for Larry should be to open his airway. Care must also be taken to protect his spine, as Larry's injuries and mechanism of injury indicate a potential spinal injury.

72. (B) After opening the airway, it may be necessary to apply gentle traction to Larry's neck to maintain spinal alignment and an adequate airway.

73. (A) At this point, administration of O_2 is indicated. Vital signs may be obtained after O_2 is begun.

74. (D) A rigid cervical collar should now be applied to protect the C-spine.

75. (C) At this time you should apply and inflate a pneumatic counterpressure device. The presence of shock takes precedence over the spinal injury. Great care should be taken to protect Larry's spine as much as possible.

76. (B) Open the airway to determine whether respirations are reestablished.

77. (B) Ventilate two times if Larry does not breathe on his own. After the two breaths, check his pulse for 5 to 10 seconds. If it is absent, start CPR. Do not administer a precordial thump.

78. (A) Your first action should always be to open the unconscious patient's airway. If respirations are not present, ventilate two times (1 1/2–2 seconds per breath). The patient poses no danger of poisoning you, as the pills have been ingested.

79. (D) CPR should be continued on Mary Ann until you are relieved by another medical person. Oftentimes, overdose or suicide patients remain alive despite their severely depressed clinical state.

80. (C) The suicide note will eventually be needed by the police, but if they are not on the scene, patient care dictates your rapid transfer of the patient and the note. The suicide note should be taken with the patient to the hospital. Do not forget to transport the pill bottles, which may enable the Emergency Department staff to determine the best course of treatment for the patient.

81. (D) The red face and ignition on but car out of gas could lead you to suspect and treat for CO poisoning. The patient may also be suffering from hypothermia. Alcohol (ETOH) intoxication is also possible. Any of the choices could be the cause for this patient's distress.

82. (C) The probable cause of the accident is alcohol intoxication. It is not uncommon for an intoxicated person to pull off the road and fall asleep with the motor running. This appears to be the case, as the ignition is still on, but the engine is not running since the car is out of fuel.

83. (A) Initial care for patients with CO poisoning is immediate evacuation from the toxic area and the administration of high-concentration O_2. After the patient is placed in the warm ambulance, vital signs can be taken.

84. (C) Until you can rule out a possible cervical injury, neck traction should be maintained on Dawn.

85. (A) Due to the long transport time, Dawn's pulseless arm should be gently straightened in an attempt to restore distal circulation. It can then be splinted by using rigid splints. Local protocol or Medical Control may direct your specific care for this type of injury.

86. (C) The normal respiratory rate for a 6-year-old child is between 20 and 25 times per minute. When in doubt, observe for signs of labored breathing, such as intercostal skin tightening and nasal flaring.

87. (D) When called to the home of a terminally ill patient, you should determine what illness exists and whether the patient and family are ready for the death. CPR is not always indicated. The family should be allowed to remain with the patient. The patient may have a DNR (Do Not Resuscitate) order signed by his physician or an Advanced Directive for Medical Care (Living Will). EMTs should be familiar with local protocols for handling such situations or contact Medical Control for patient care instructions.

88. (B) The signs and symptoms of an acute CVA (stroke) include paralysis on one side of the body, drooling, and an elevated blood pressure. The pulse rate may be slow.

89. (D) The stroke patient requires very gentle handling. He should be transported on his affected side to prevent aspiration. Although the patient may appear unconscious, he may be aware of all that is happening around him. A respiratory rate of 10 or above should be sufficient to adequately ventilate the patient. The airway must be monitored constantly. Nitroglycerin is used to relieve chest pain; therefore, it is not indicated in this situation.

90. (A) Not uncommon are the so-called "mystery crashes" that have no apparent explanation. You should provide the basic ABCs to this patient and suspect a possible acute MI, CVA, or pulmonary embolism.

Critical Questions

A wide range of topics are covered by the questions in this review manual. Some questions test your knowledge of basic information while others determine your grasp of proper procedures and their sequence. Furthermore, certain questions require that you apply information or theory to a new problem. Within the framework of each chapter, specific questions focus on critical material that you should understand thoroughly.

The author has selected questions in each chapter which he has designated as "critical," and which are listed in the table below. Check whether you have answered these questions correctly. If you have missed a substantial number, it may indicate certain weaknesses in your knowledge base and point you to sources which you can study further. This book's bibliography lists the main EMT textbooks which explain in detail the background data for all the questions.

Critical Questions by Chapter

Chapter	Critical Questions
2. Roles and Responsibilities of the EMT	6, 10, 15, 17, 19, 23
3. Personal Safety	1, 4, 5, 6, 7, 8, 13, 16
4. Anatomy, Physiology, and Diagnostic Signs	6, 15, 16, 18, 19, 20, 26, 32, 34, 36, 37, 38, 41, 42, 46, 58, 66, 71

5. Respiratory and Circulatory Systems 2, 3, 4, 11, 5, 17, 20, 26, 28, 27, 30, 32, 35, 36, 37, 41, 42, 44, 48, 50, 51, 56, 57, 60, 63, 65, 67, 71, 73, 77, 85, 98, 102, 108, 109, 112, 113, 116

6. Wounds, Bleeding, and Shock 1, 2, 3, 8, 17, 19, 20, 23, 24, 30, 34, 36, 37, 46, 48, 50, 51, 52, 58, 59, 66, 78, 81, 83, 85, 89

7. Musculoskeletal System 6, 7, 11, 13, 14, 20, 21, 28, 38, 41, 42, 44, 48, 50, 57

8. Nervous System and Head Injuries 1, 2, 8, 12, 17, 22, 25, 33

9. Chest, Abdominal and Genital Injuries 3, 5, 7, 9, 11, 15, 17, 27, 32, 38, 39

10. Medical Emergencies 5, 7, 10, 11, 18, 20, 24, 25, 26, 33, 38, 41, 46, 52, 53, 55, 66, 69

11. Pediatric Emergencies and Childbirth 4, 5, 6, 9, 17, 21, 24, 30, 38, 42, 43

12. Environmental Injury Emergencies 1, 4, 7, 11, 12, 13, 23, 34, 35, 36, 38, 39, 41

13. Behavioral Problems 6, 8, 14, 16, 17, 19, 24

14. Transportation, Patient Handling, and Scene Management 2, 4, 5, 7, 12, 16, 23, 30, 32

15. Situational Reviews 2, 8, 18, 20, 21, 23, 30, 41, 44, 53, 58, 66, 69, 81, 87, 88

Bibliography

American Academy of Orthopaedic Surgeons. *Emergency Care and Transportation of the Sick and Injured*. 5th Ed. Chicago: American Academy of Orthopaedic Surgeons, 1992.

Bunting-Blake, Linda, et al. *Defibrillation, a Manual for the EMT*. 1st Ed. Philadelphia: J. B. Lippincott Company, 1986.

Campbell, John E. *Basic Trauma Life Support—Advanced*. 2nd Ed. Englewood Cliffs: Brady, a Regents/Prentice Hall Division, 1988.

Caroline, Nancy L. *Emergency Care in the Streets*. 4th Ed. Boston: Little, Brown and Company, 1991.

Caroline, Nancy L. *Emergency Medical Treatment*. 3rd Ed. Boston: Little, Brown and Company, 1991.

Champion, H. R., et al. "Trauma Score." *Critical Care Medicine* 9(9) 672–676, 1981.

Childs, Bradford J., and Donald J. Ptacnik. *Emergency Ambulance Driving*. 1st Ed. Englewood Cliffs: Brady, a Regents/Prentice Hall Division, 1986.

Dernocoeur, Kate Boyd. *Streetsense: Communication, Safety, and Control*. 2nd Ed. Englewood Cliffs: Brady, a Regents/Prentice Hall Division, 1990.

Emergency Cardiac Care Committee and Subcommittees, American Heart Association. Guidelines for Cardiopulmonary Resuscitation and Emergency Cardiac Care. *The Journal of the American Medical Association* 1992; 268: 2171–2302.

Grant, Harvey D., Murray, Jr., R. H., and J. David Bergeron. *Emergency Care*. 5th Ed. Englewood Cliffs: Brady, a Regents/Prentice Hall Division, 1990.

Gray, Henry, FRS. *Gray's Anatomy*. 29th printing. Philadelphia: Running Press, 1974.

Hafen, Brent Q., and Keith J. Karren. *Prehospital Emergency Care & Crisis Intervention*. 4th Ed. Englewood Cliffs: Brady, a Regents/Prentice Hall Division, 1992.

Henry, Mark C., MD, and Edward R. Stapleton, EMT-P. *EMT Prehospital Care*. 1st Ed. Philadelphia: W. B. Saunders Company, 1992.

Jones, Shirley A., MS Ed, MHA, EMT-P, et al. *Advanced Emergency Care for Paramedic Practice*. 1st Ed. Philadelphia: J. B. Lippincott Company, 1992.

Lillis, Carol A. *Brady's Introduction to Medical Terminology*. 1st Ed. Englewood Cliffs: Brady, a Regents/Prentice Hall Division, 1983.

Moore, Ronald E. *Vehicle Rescue and Extrication*. 1st Ed. St. Louis: Mosby-Year Book, Inc., 1991.

Phillips, Charles, MD. *Basic Life Support Skills Manual*. 2nd Ed. Englewood Cliffs: Brady, a Regents/Prentice Hall Division, 1986.

Pre-Hospital Trauma Life Support Committee of the National Association of Emergency Medical Technicians. *Pre-Hospital Trauma Life Support*. 1st Ed. Akron: Emergency Training, 1986.

Rescue Training Associates. *Action Guide for Emergency Service Personnel*. 1st Ed. Englewood Cliffs: Brady, a Regents/Prentice Hall Division, 1985.

Stults, Kenneth. *EMT-D Prehospital Defibrillation*. 1st Ed. Englewood Cliffs: Brady, a Regents/Prentice Hall Division, 1986.

U.S. Department of Health and Human Services. *EMS and the Hearing Impaired*. 1st Ed. Rockville, MD: U.S. Department of Health and Human Services, Public Health Service/Health Services Administration, 1981.

U.S. Department of Transportation. *Air Medical Crew National Standard Curriculum—Basic Student Manual*. 1st Ed. Pasadena: ASHBEAMS, 1988.

U.S. Department of Transportation. *Basic Training Course/Emergency Medical Technician: Instructor's Lesson Plans*. 3rd Ed. Washington, DC: U.S. Department of Transportation, National Highway Traffic Safety Administration, 1984.

U.S. Fire Administration. *Guide to Developing and Managing an Emergency Service Infection Control Program*. 1st Ed. Emmitsburg, MD: United States Fire Administration, 1992.